Gudrun Bornhöft, Peter F. Matthiessen (eds)

Homeopathy in Healthcare –
Effectiveness, Appropriateness, Safety, Costs

Gudrun Bornhöft, Peter F. Matthiessen (eds)

Homeopathy in Healthcare – Effectiveness, Appropriateness, Safety, Costs

An HTA report on homeopathy as part of the Swiss Complementary Medicine Evaluation Programme

Translated from the German by Margot M. Saar

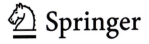 Springer

Prof. Peter F. Matthiessen
Zentrum für Integrative Medizin der
Universität Witten/Herdecke gGmbH
Gerhard-Kienle-Weg 6
58313 Herdecke, Germany

Dr. med. Gudrun Bornhöft
Reußstr. 1
38640 Goslar, Germany

ISBN-13   978-3-642-20638-2 Springer-Verlag Berlin Heidelberg New York

Bibliographic information Deutsche Bibliothek
The Deutsche Bibliothek lists this publication in Deutsche Nationalbibliographie;
detailed bibliographic data is available in the internet at <http://dnb.ddb.de>.

SpringerMedizin
Springer-Verlag GmbH
ein Unternehmen von Springer Science+Business
springer.de

Planning: Diana Kraplow
Project management: Diana Kraplow
Copy-Editing: Mary Schäfer, Buchen-Hettingen

Translated into English from the German, Margot M. Saar

Cover design: deblik Berlin
Typesetting and reproduction of the figures:
Fotosatz-Service Köhler GmbH – Reinhold Schöberl, Würzburg

18/5141 – 5 4 3 2 1 0   SPIN 80052924

Table of Contents

Introduction

Peter F. Matthiessen, Gudrun Bornhöft

The present HTA report on homeopathy, now published in book format, was part of the 'Complementary Medicine Evaluation Programme' (PEK[1]) which was set up following a decision by the Swiss government in 1998 to 'provisionally' include the complementary medical disciplines – anthroposophic medicine, homeopathy, traditional Chinese medicine, phytotherapy and neural therapy – in the list of services covered by the national statutory health insurance.

HTA is short for Health Technology Assessment, an established scientific procedure which, in contrast to the meta-analyses and systematic reviews specified by the Cochrane Collaboration Standards, examines not only the efficacy of a particular intervention, but especially also its 'real-world effectiveness', its appropriateness, safety and economy. HTAs are therefore much wider in scope and politically more informative. They include material that is 'normally' not taken into consideration, such as observational studies, good case series and longitudinal cohort studies.

The specialities named were to be examined for their real-world effectiveness, appropriateness and cost-effectiveness, and the result was intended to inform the decision regarding their future within primary health care (cf. Chap. 2 of this book and Wolf 2006).

The motivation for the project and how it evolved reflect the polarities and diverging streams that are now ubiquitous in many countries with regard to complementary and alternative medicines (CAM) while also elucidating institutional processes:

The PEK programme was prompted by the high demand and widespread use and acceptance of complementary medical treatment, as well as by the political hope for its economic and preventive use. At the same time, mainstream medicine frequently expressed its concern that complementary medical treatment was ineffective, if not harmful. The question was: how could one arrive at a decision that would satisfy society while meeting the requirements of scientific medicine?

Following a 5-year preparation phase, the evaluation project was split into a practical component (field study), as part of which special trials were conducted on parameters relevant for practitioners and patients, and a literary component (HTA reports) to assess international publications for evidence of the (real-world) effectiveness, appropriateness, safety and economy of the treatments. The latter was extended by a smaller sub-project that encompassed a quantitative analysis of the quality of clinical trials in the CAM disciplines mentioned above compared with those of conventional medicine.

After the above-mentioned 5-year preparation phase, less than 2 years remained for the completion of the projects.

Before the overall project was finalized, the results of the smaller quantitative sub-study, which – contrary to the implicit intention of an HTA – had evaluated only experimental trials (randomized double-blind trials), became known out of context. While the overall conclusion was that studies of homeopathy and phytotherapy were of better quality than comparable studies of conventional medicine, the subsidiary meta-analysis of the qualitatively best trials (according to internal validity criteria) demonstrated efficacy for the interventions of conventional medicine and phytotherapy but no significant difference to placebo for homeopathic treatment. (Concerning the problem of reducing qualitative evaluations to purely internally valid criteria cf. Chaps. 5 and 13.)

The 'negative result' for homeopathy caused a massive furore prior to conclusion of the PEK project and following its subsequent publication (Shang et al. 2005), culminating in the unfortunately titled Lancet editorial 'The end of homeopathy' (editorial 2005).

---

1   PEK – Programm Evaluation Komplementärmedizin

In contrast to this subsidiary result, which was of little relevance for the political decision, the much more comprehensive and differentiated HTAs ascertained **that the individual CAM interventions,** especially homeopathy, **were effective, under Swiss conditions safe and, as far as could be judged from the trial situation, also cost-efficient.**

In their overall assessment the PEK review committee attested good quality and replicable results with scientifically tenable conclusions to the HTAs on anthroposophic medicine, homeopathy, phytotherapy and TCM phytotherapy. The editorial of the journal *Forschende Komplementärmedizin* (Walach and Heusser 2006), which published short versions of the HTAs on homeopathy (Bornhöft et al. 2006), anthroposophic medicine (Kienle et al. 2006) and traditional Chinese medicine (Maxion-Bergemann et al. 2006), speaks of high, partly even highest, quality also because 'the model validities of individual studies, such as in the field of homeopathy, were never before [...] so critically and constructively integrated in the evaluation results'. It emphasizes that the HTA reports of the PEK project underwent a multi-stage quality assurance procedure, which means that the quality of their information can be regarded as scientifically confirmed. Walach and Heusser consider the PEK's HTA reports to be fundamentally of higher value than reviews of experimental studies, including the above-mentioned meta-analyses. With regard to the further political decision process they report: 'It will also not be concealed that the evaluation committee employed by the Swiss Federal Office of Public Health (FOPH) for the overall assessment of the PEK results recommended in its final report that anthroposophic medicine, homeopathy and phytotherapy, on the basis of their documented utility, should continue to be covered by the statutory health insurance. Under pressure from the authorities, however, this recommendation was removed from the final version of the report, and in June 2005 Federal Councillor Pascal Couchepin excluded complementary medical services by physicians from the statutory health insurance scheme.'

The present, corrected and partly revised book picks up the controversies of the discussion on methods. It especially re-evaluates Shang et al.'s (2005) quantitative analysis, taking into consideration criteria of external and model validity as well as of internal validity – with a truly remarkable result in favour of homeopathy – and adds it to the original text (Chap. 5). The chapter also throws light on the field of tension between an 'objective' and strongly formalized evaluation by investigators who are not specialists in the given field and the replicability of the subjectively generated empirical knowledge of practising physicians, and their respective strengths and weaknesses.

Further changes to the 2004 version include a restructuring of the result presentations in Chaps. 7 and 10, in-depth discussions (Chap. 13) and the subdivision of the HTA into individual chapters with allocation of authors.

Acknowledgements

We would like to thank all those who made the revision and publication of this book possible, in particular the PanMedion Foundation Zurich.

References

Bornhöft G, Wolf U, Ammon K, Righetti M, Maxion-Bergemann S, Baumgartner S, Thurneysen AE, Matthiessen PF (2006) Effectiveness, safety and cost-effectiveness of homeopathy in general practice – summarized health technology assessment. Forschende Komplementärmedizin 13 [Suppl 2]:19–29

Editorial (2005) The end of homeopathy. Lancet 366:690; DOI:10.1016/S0140-6736(05)67149-8

Kienle GS, Kiene H, Albonico HU (2006) Anthroposophische Medizin: Health Technology Assessment Bericht – Kurzfassung. Forschende Komplementärmedizin 13 [Suppl 2]:7–18

Maxion-Bergemann S, Wolf M, Bornhöft G, Matthiessen PF, Wolf U (2006) Complementary and alternative medicine costs – a systematic literature review. Forschende Komplementärmedizin 13 [Suppl 2]:42–45

Shang A, Huwiler-Muntener K, Nartey L, Jüni P, Dörig S, Sterne JAC, Pewsner D, Egger M (2005) Are the clinical effects of homeopathy placebo effects? Comparative study of placebo-controlled trials of homeopathy and allopathy. Lancet 366:726–732

Walach H, Heusser P (2006) Effektiv oder nicht? Entscheiden Sie selbst! – Die PEK-HTA-Berichte. Forschende Komplementärmedizin 13 [Suppl 2]:2–3

Wolf U (2006) Die HTA-Berichte und ihre Bedeutung für die Komplementärmedizin. Forschende Komplementärmedizin 13 [Suppl 2]:1

Background and objectives of HTA

Stefanie Maxion-Bergemann, Gudrun Bornhöft

2.1   Background

On 9 July 1998 the Swiss government decided to include the five most important complementary medical disciplines – anthroposophic medicine, homeopathy, neural therapy, phytotherapy and traditional Chinese medicine (TCM, Chinese phytotherapy in particular) – into the list of services covered by the Swiss statutory health insurance (KLV[1]). As a precondition for reimbursement the physician consulted had to be fully qualified and the time of coverage was limited to the period leading up to 30 June 2005. During this period, an evaluation of the specialities mentioned with regard to their 'effectiveness, appropriateness and economy' was to be prepared and put into practice as from 2003.

For the evaluation phase a group of experts set up the 'Complementary Medicine Evaluation Programme' with two components: one was practical (Swiss Patient Care Evaluation Study in Complementary Medicine, SPEC) and the other was a literature study.

From the homeopathic side it was reported that as a first step in the PEK programme comprehensive reviewing and stock-taking of homeopathic research had been planned and agreed upon. The HTA report then commissioned focused, however – in line with the customary HTA concept – on a different selection of literature, with the result that a comprehensive review of homeopathic research is still outstanding.

The 'literature' sub-project had two parts: 1) five individual HTA[2] reports were put together, namely for anthroposophic medicine, homeopathy, neural therapy, phytotherapy and traditional Chinese medicine (phytotherapy); 2) the Institute for social and preventive medicine (ISPM[3]) at Berne University, Switzerland, prepared meta-analyses on RCTs in homeopathy, TCM and phytotherapy.

Based on the documentation arising from the field study, HTA reports and meta-analyses, the specialist associations submitted an application, in 2005, to the Swiss Federal Commission for General Health Insurance (ELK[4]), the institution that was to decide whether homeopathy was to remain part of the basic health-care provision.

The HTA reports were commissioned by the Swiss Federal Social Insurance Office (FSIO)[5] and jointly compiled by the PanMedion Foundation Zurich, the Chair of Medical Theory and Complementary Medicine at the University of Witten/Herdecke (Germany) and the Institute for Applied Epistemology and Medical Methodology (IFAEMM[6]) from January 2003 to August 2004.

Structure and content of the HTA reports were based on K. Linde's application documents, which had been prepared before the reports were commissioned. Form and content of the reports are clearly specified in the application documents. These documents have mostly been adhered to, with a few helpful additions in some places. It was known before the project began that the individual medical specialities each possessed characteristic properties that needed to be taken into account. Some aspects are described in the next section.

---

1   KLV – Krankenpflege Leistungsverordnung
2   HTA – Health Technology Assessment
3   ISPM – Institut für Sozial- und Präventivmedizin
4   ELK – Eidgenössische Kommission für allgemeine Leistungen
5   BSV – Bundesamt für Sozialversicherung
6   IFAEMM – Institut für angewandte Erkenntnistheorie und medizinische Methodologie

2.2 **Objectives**

1. Review of publications
   - What kinds and quantities of scientific publications are available for the respective medical speciality via online databases (libraries)?
2. The situation in Switzerland / general parameters
   - What parameters, legal and otherwise, apply to the respective medical speciality in Switzerland?
   - What infrastructure is in place for the use of the respective medical speciality and the supply of medicines?
   - What particular problems arise from these parameters?
3. What is the current state of (preclinical) research?
4. Effectiveness
   What evidence of effectiveness is available with regard to
   - the speciality in general, based on published systematic reviews and meta-analyses?
   - one chosen indication, based on published studies of different design?
5. Appropriateness/safety
   - What kinds and incidences of possible unexpected adverse effects are described?
   - What are the legal regulations with regard to the safety of the medicines?
   - How are training and further training structured to ensure safety of application?
6. Appropriateness/demand (use)
   - Which physicians apply the speciality in Switzerland and in what way?
   - Which complementary medical methods are used or applied how often by which patients?
   - Why are they used and what level of effectiveness is being observed?
   - What is the situation in Switzerland?
   - What is the situation in Europe and the USA?
7. Economy
   - What research into the cost-effectiveness of the methods is available from Switzerland and elsewhere; how valid is it and what are its conclusions?

Introduction to the speciality of homeopathy – principles and definition

Marco Righetti, Klaus v. Ammon, Peter Mattmann, André Thurneysen

3.1   Preface

The characteristic features of homeopathy are its particular drug therapy and application, its drug provings on the healthy subject, the development of its pharmacology, the case-taking and exact observation of the individual patient's symptoms and idiosyncrasies, the conclusions drawn from numerous individual healing processes and its extended treatment target. All these aspects result in an approach that is fundamentally different, in theory and practice, from mainstream medicine. While both systems are based on exact empirical observation, their methods of observation and interpretation differ. In mainstream medicine, treatment is based on the clinical diagnosis while the symptoms displayed by the individual patient play a lesser role. In homeopathy, on the other hand, the choice of medication depends on the totality of symptoms and signs displayed by the individual patient. The clinical diagnosis is important for assessing the medical situation but has little bearing on the choice of remedy. Administering homeopathic remedies and mixtures merely on the basis of a clinical diagnosis goes against the principles of homeopathy.

A short outline of the history of homeopathy (based, among others, on Hahnemann 1828, 1835, 1842; Haehl 1922; Seiler 1988) will introduce the special aspects of the homeopathic method.

3.2   The principle of similarity or 'Law of Similars'

In 1796, following his drug provings on healthy persons, Samuel Hahnemann (1755–1843) pronounced the principle of similarity: *similia similibus curentur* (may like be cured by like). With these famous words homeopathy was born as a scientific approach to healing, initially as a working hypothesis. Since then, the understanding of the similarity principle has evolved and been deepened. Homeopathy's defining principle states that a disease is cured by the remedy whose drug picture is most similar to the disease picture. 'Similarity' means an essential congruence that is manifest in the totality of characteristic symptoms and signs apparent in the patient.

Looking at reality in terms of similarities is unfamiliar to our mostly linear, causal-analytical thinking, although the approach goes back to Hippocrates and Paracelsus. For Hahnemann, a scientific, rational drug therapy could not possibly rest on ever-changing theories, but solely on meticulous observation and experience. This empirical-inductive method (i.e. drawing conclusions from observation and experience rather than 'deducing' them from existent theories) made Hahnemann one of the first scientists in the medical field.

3.3   Homeopathic pharmacology

Since then, countless drug provings on healthy subjects and toxicological studies have promoted the expansion of homeopathic pharmacology. The most important evidence still arises from practical clinical experience and from the successful treatment of millions of patients. The homeopathic Materia Medica has by now grown to include more than 1000 remedies.

3.4 The homeopathic examination and remedy selection

The homeopathic examination (case-taking) differs in method and objectives from that of conventional medicine. With the latter, treatment is determined by the clinical diagnosis which, in homeopathy, is of importance for assessing the medical situation but not for the choice of remedy. The decisive factor when selecting a medicine in homeopathy is the phenomenological assessment of the totality of a patient's individual, characteristic and conspicuous symptoms, signs and idiosyncrasies. Homeopathy sees in the individual symptoms externally perceptible manifestations (*gestalt*) of an internal, not observable process (referred to as illness, 'regulatory disturbance', 'disturbance of the vital force' by Hahnemann).

In practice, the differentiation between acute and chronic disease can be relevant in some cases. With acute conditions that need treatment, the conspicuous, acute symptoms of the individual case can determine the choice of medicine. With a chronic disorder it is necessary to meticulously assess the entire disease process, including previous outbreaks, so that the right constitutional remedy can be found. Homeopaths often try to treat acute disease with the chronic constitutional remedy. A full case-taking session can last several hours, depending on the complexity of the problem and the homeopath's approach.

Case-taking is followed by evaluation and a remedy search, which happens in two stages: (a) Repertorisation, i.e. selection, appraisal and scaling of the symptoms with the help of symptom manuals (repertories) that list symptom patterns and the corresponding known remedies by organ and body area. (b) Differential diagnosis and remedy selection by means of a case study in which the patient's symptoms and signs are compared with potential remedies from the Materia Medica and the remedy (*simillimum*) is selected that comes closest to the respective patient's condition.

With chronic disease the initial examination is particularly long. It is often not possible to find the most suitable remedy immediately; sometimes it cannot be found at all. Selection is particularly difficult and therefore more time-consuming with the hardly researched and little known 'small remedies' and in complex cases, where various remedies have to be tried in succession.

In rare cases the individualisation principle can be restricted, when there is an obvious external cause (traumatology, insect bites etc.), for instance, an epidemic or individual local symptoms. With most disease processes it fully applies, however.

What has been said so far illustrates why it is possible to treat three totally different conditions (in the conventional medical sense) such as recurrent purulent pharyngitis, hay fever and migraine in one patient with a single, individually chosen chronic constitutional remedy because there is only one chronic condition, only one patient who suffers from it. It is possible, on the other hand, that two patients who present with totally different clinical symptoms require the same homeopathic remedy because their individual symptoms are similar.

3.5 Medicines: their manufacture, application and mode of action

Homeopathic medicines are manufactured in a particular way. The raw materials used originate from plants, minerals and animals (also animal and disease products) which are processed in a special way (potentisation): the substances are continuously diluted in decimal and centesimal stages; solids are triturated with lactose and liquids are succussed in a water-alcohol solution. Decimal potencies (D) are diluted at each stage at a ratio of 1:10, centesimal potencies (C) at 1:100. The 50,000 dilutions (Q or LM potencies) constitute a special variety. The potentisation process is the result of continuous experience and observation of patient reactions. The fact that ever higher potencies were used in the history of homeopathy was a frequent bone of contention. From a conventional pharmacological point of view a medicinal effect seems most improbable, as according to Avogadro's number, no molecule of the medicinal substance will be left in the solution from the 24th decimal or 12th centesimal potency.

The dilutions' mode of action requires a homeopathic explanation. Homeopathic remedies are backed by 200 years of empirical observation of millions of patients which shows that high potencies are often particularly effective if they are optimally matched to the patient's individual symptom picture. The mode of action of homeopathic remedies cannot be demonstrated with modern scientific methods. Due to a misapplied positivism that sees the reality of nature merely as the sum total of its measurable and quantifiable phenomena, a 'lack of evidence' is often seen to mean the same as 'lack of effectiveness'. Negative preconceptions regarding homeopathy are widespread, and its effects are said to be placebo effects.

What is overdue is a scientific approach that looks more thoroughly at the observed phenomena and at how they contradict the fundamental tenets of the dominant scientific system. The inflexibility of the prevailing scientific paradigm has long been known to, and revised by, epistemological science. The current thinking and research of mainstream medicine are influenced mainly by Newton's mechanistic and strictly causal-analytical physics (classical reductionist biomedical model), which ignores the more complex phenomena of nature, the organism's systemic correlations, its life processes and overall regulation, and life as a whole, as well as qualitative experiences and the phenomena of spiritual science. Modern physics with its theory of relativity and quantum physics has long overtaken Newtonian mechanics and is paving the way for an understanding of the homeopathic mechanism of action.

Research into the natural and possibly also spiritual scientific phenomena that underlie the biological systems is still in its very early stages. Despite the problem with measurability, unexpected and inexplicable changes have been observed in recent years in physical-chemical experiments with potentized solutions, even though it has not yet been possible to present hard scientific evidence. Potentized remedies certainly comply with wave and quantum physics, the results of cluster research, and the chemistry of solids, as well as with modern chaos theory. On the basis of this, a mode of action that is conveyed by specific electromagnetic, energetic and structural changes in the potentized solution is conceivable; but homeopathic phenomena might well rest on processes that cannot be ascertained by natural science.

Dosage and administration of remedies are also special in homeopathy, with smallest doses often being given in a totally individualized way.

3.6 The concept of disease in homeopathy and conventional medicine

Despite his successful treatment of acute diseases, Hahnemann often found that an underlying chronic disease continued to gradually progress. While conventional medicine today regards and treats disease as a local or biochemical disorder, Hahnemann looked beyond the local, momentary manifestations to the chronic disease process of the entire organism. The importance of the chronic disease doctrine lies in the observation of chronic disease processes and in establishing the suitable treatment.

From the homeopathic point of view, the disease itself consists in a regulatory disturbance of the organism. It cannot be observed directly, but only via the sum total of its externally perceptible symptoms and signs. Exact observation and evaluation of the totality of individual symptoms leads to the selection of the individual single remedy that is able to restore balance to the patient's organism. Homeopathy is therefore a regulatory therapy. In homeopathy, healing does not mean eliminating individual symptoms, as in conventional medicine, but eliminating all disease symptoms including the susceptibility in chronic cases and restoring the patient's mental and physical equilibrium. This view brings homeopathy close to the modern system-theoretical disease models.

The vital force, just as vitality in general, cannot be measured and quantified by science, but it exists as a phenomenon. Although homeopathy cannot explain these fundamental properties of the organism either, it can observe them phenomenologically and try to describe and treat them.

3.7   Indications and limitations of homeopathy

Many acute and chronic conditions, especially in primary health care, can be treated homeopathically as long as the patient's regulatory and self-healing powers ('vital force') can still be adequately stimulated. The success rate varies depending on the complexity and severity of the individual case and the most suitable medicine.

Obvious limitations exist where there is a compelling indication for substitution therapy (such as insulin for juvenile diabetes) or surgical intervention (with bone fractures, for instance), or with severe terminal pathologies where regulation is no longer possible. From the homeopathic point of view, surgical intervention is not always necessarily indicated and even with severe pathologies cost-effective and side-effect-free palliation and alleviation are possible. Additional (dietary, psycho-social) measures are also included in the homeopathic approach.

3.8   Other therapies known as homeopathy

Next to classical homeopathy, which proceeds in the way described and uses only single remedies, there are other approaches referred to as homeopathy which are only partly homeopathic or not at all. Organotropic homeopathy does not rely on individualisation and exact observation to the same extent, and remedies are often selected on the basis of clinical or 'proven indications' ('clinical homeopathy'). Isopathy homeopathically processes and applies substances that induce disease symptoms, such as pollen allergens for hay fever. 'Complex homeopathy' is still very popular with pharmacists and practitioners and for self-medication. It uses mixed remedies in mostly low potencies (mixed or combination preparations) for particular conventionally established symptoms and diseases. These methods present a contradiction in themselves and are not consistent with the fundamental tenets of homeopathy (similarity principle, observation of the totality of symptoms, individualisation, single remedy selection). In rare cases and when used for the short term such mixtures may well serve to alleviate less severe acute conditions. In the long-term or with more frequent application they can blur the symptom picture, induce drug-proving symptoms and render any subsequent classical homeopathic treatment more difficult.

3.9   Homeopathy research

For details concerning the research problems and outcomes see Chap. 4 as well as Righetti (1988) and Halter/ Righetti (1998/99).

3.10   References

Blackie M (1990)Lebendige Homöopathie. Sonntag, Munich
Braun A (1995) Methodik der Homöotherapie. Sonntag, Stuttgart
Genneper T, Wegener A (2001)Lehrbuch der Homöopathie. Haug, Heidelberg
Gumpert M (1989) Hahnemann, 2nd edn. Aurum, Freiburg i. Br.
Gypser KH (1995) Wissenswertes für Patienten über Homöopathie. Haug, Heidelberg
Haehl R (1925) Samuel Hahnemann (biography), 2 vols. Schwabe, Leipzig
Hahnemann S (1983) Die chronischen Krankheiten, theoretischer Teil (1828). Haug, Heidelberg
Hahnemann S(1999) Organon der Heilkunst (1842). Haug, Heidelberg
Halter K, Righetti M (1998) Klassische Homöopathie (parts 1–3). Zum Nachweis von Wirksamkeit und Nutzen einer komplementärmedizinischen Methode. Schweizerische Zeitschrift für Ganzheitsmedizin. 10:252–257, 343–346 und (1999) 11:1
Illing KH (1988) Homöopathie für Anfänger (introduction), Homöopathische Taschenbücher vol 1. Haug, Heidelberg
Kent JT (2002) Repertory of the Homeopathic Materia Medica (6th American edn, reprint). Jain Publishers, Delhi
Köhler G (1993) Lehrbuch der Homöopathie, vol 1. Grundlagen und Anwendung. Hippokrates, Stuttgart
Meili W (1989) Grundkurs in klassischer Homöopathie. Sonntag, Regensburg
Righetti M (1988) Forschung in der Homöopathie; Grundlagen, Problematik und Ergebnisse. Burgdorf, Göttingen
Schroyens F (1993) Synthesis Repertorium. Homeopathic Book Publishers, London
Seiler H (1988) Die Entwicklung von Samuel Hahnemanns ärztlicher Praxis anhand ausgewählter Krankengeschichten. Haug, Heidelberg
Stumpf W (1990) Homöopathie. Gräfe und Unzer, Munich
Van Zandvoort R (1994) The complete repertory. IRHIS-Verlag, Leidschendamm
Vithoulkas G (1986) Die wissenschaftliche Homöopathie. Burgdorf, Göttingen
Voegeli A (1993) Die korrekte homöopathische Behandlung in der täglichen Praxis, 10th edn. Heidelberg: Haug,
Wright-Hubbard E (1993) Kurzlehrgang der Homöopathie, 2nd edn. Barthel & Barthel, Berg

Homeopathy: Research and Research Problems (preclinical and clinical)

Marco Righetti, Stephan Baumgartner, Klaus v. Ammon

4.1   Introduction and Research Problems

The discussion of the problems and value of homeopathy presupposes a thorough knowledge of its scientific foundations. The fundamental difference between conventional medicine and homeopathy requires the employment of different research tools. While both systems rely on exact empirical observation, their methodologies and pharmacologies differ in the way their medicines are manufactured, in their modes of observation and treatment and in their therapeutic objectives.

For an adequate evaluation of the literature available today and for the assessment of the effectiveness, appropriateness and economy of homeopathy, the following facts need to be taken into account: 200 years of experience with a vast number of patients, numerous case reports in the literature, unexplored material available in homeopathic practices and reports about successful treatment in large-scale epidemics have never been systematically and scientifically researched. The most recent in-depth surveys go back to the late 1980s and were conducted by Walach 1986, Poitevin 1987 and Righetti 1988. In recent years, only selective surveys (Kleijnen et al. 1991, Boissel et al. 1996, Walach et al. 1997, Linde et al. 1997, Clausius 1998, Linde & Melchart 1998, Ernst 1999, Cucherat et al. 2000, Wein 2002, Mathie 2003 and Dean 2004) have been published, along with a number of papers relating to specific indications.

To what extent the systemized experience from particular periods of time is being considered as 'soft' empirical facts in the scientific and public debate is not primarily a question of scientific research but mostly an epistemological question with political and social dimensions.

Homeopathy has its own particular research tradition and has always relied on empirical research. Its system-immanent research includes drug provings on the healthy subject, the exact phenomenological observation of symptoms and reactions, the individualized treatment of the patient on the basis of the similarity principle, evaluation of the healing processes, and observation of numerous individual cases and – in epidemics – collectives as well as its special drug manufacturing techniques. From the point of view of homeopathy, this is the only kind of research that is relevant to its practice. The results of the empirical observation which determines the quality of the homeopathic treatment can be found in the homeopathic Materia Medica, in the symptom manuals that are based on it (repertories) and in its rules of dosage and application.

Leaning on its own philosophy and research system, conventional medicine often displays a sceptical and dismissive attitude towards this kind of research and its results and insists on randomized, controlled, double-blind trials as clinical proof of efficacy. This approach is seen as controversial even within evidence-based medicine, especially when applied to complex systems such as psychotherapy and homeopathy.

Many experimental and clinical trials that were based on the methods of conventional medicine have been carried out in homeopathy over the past decades with a view to gaining scientific and political recognition. From a homeopathic point of view, it was justification research more than anything else and did not provide any new insights into homeopathy as such. Homeopathy experts continue to claim that the great majority of existing homeopathy trials were conducted with inadequate means, that their designs ignore essential principles of homeopathy and thus increase the likelihood of false-negative results. The trials have almost nothing in common with the actual practice of homeopathy in Switzerland; their external and model validities are very low (cf. Chap. 5). The proponents of homeopathy point out that research results thus obtained, even though significant in the pharmacotherapy of conventional medicine, are of little relevance to homeopathic practice and therefore hardly known among homeopaths! Only if these considerations, including the fundamental difference between allopathic and homeopathic thinking, are taken into account, will it make any sense to interpret the research results attained by conventional medical methods; this fact is ignored by many representatives of conventional medical science and also by some homeopathic scientists. Homeopathy is nevertheless interested in experimental and clinical studies because, if these actually took into account the conditions that are specific to homeopathy, they could promote knowledge acquisition in homeopathy and provide exemplary evidence that (highly) potentized remedies, if applied with strict adherence to recognized methods, bring about a specific effect or action.

The following outline of important experimental evidence of effectiveness and clinical efficacy is not complete due to space restrictions and to the fact that the recently published general surveys are still rudimentary.

4.2 Preclinical Research

Homeopathy relies primarily on the observation of healthy and diseased *human beings*. The 'pillars' of homeopathy such as the simile principle, drug provings on the healthy, and the idea of potentising medicinal substances arose from this fundamental precept.

Preclinical research (on animals, plants, and cells as well as purely physical structure investigations) can therefore not be seen as *homeopathic in the true sense*. This is also apparent from the questions typically investigated, which relate to general scientific problems rather than aspects that are specific to homeopathy:

- Do highly diluted remedies (potencies) also show a specific effect in other living organisms (such as plants or animals)?
- Do homeopathic potencies have a specific physico-chemical structure?

Preclinical investigations of this kind were initially carried out by proponents of homeopathy as 'justification research' in order to demonstrate its specific effectiveness to 'official' science. Fundamental research is now increasingly conducted by university institutes out of general scientific interest, and also by homeopathic pharmacists for quality-assurance purposes.

When evaluating the outcomes of preclinical research one must therefore keep in mind that it practically ignores two of the three main pillars of homeopathy (drug proving on the healthy subject and the simile principle) and that these cannot be assessed through preclinical investigation (problem of non-transferability to human beings); the primary focus of fundamental research has always been the potentisation principle.

4.2.1 Fundamental physico-chemical research

From the 1950s on, experimental physico-chemical research has concentrated on the question of whether a specific material structure of homeopathic vehicles (water, alcohol, lactose) can be demonstrated, based on the prevalent pharmacological view that recognizes as specific medicinal effects solely those of (sufficiently highly concentrated) materially present substances on human cells.

The process of evaluating the older literature has only just begun (for surveys cf. Becker-Witt et al. 2003 and Weingärtner 1992, 2002). More recent investigations with NMR or UV spectroscopy as well as electrochemical thermodynamic measurements suggest a dynamisation of the solvent structure for homeopathic potencies compared with controls (cf. Demangeat et al. 2004, Elia and Niccoli 2000), which means that homeopathic potentisation most probably involves a principle of action that is different from the 'usually' assumed molecular, often receptor-mediated, modes of drug action.

Processes that are purely regulatory and/or involve the transmission of energetic information and cannot yet be ascertained by contemporary physical measuring methods are also being considered.

4.2.2 Botanical studies

From the 1920s to the present, plants have been used to examine the homeopathic potentisation procedure with a view to discovering whether specific actions of homeopathic potencies can also be observed in plants and whether, with the help of such examinations, fundamental properties of homeopathic dilutions can be established.

Observations by various researchers seem to confirm this. The literature available in this field has not yet been sufficiently explored (e.g. Vickers 1999 and Baumgartner et al. 2000), but some conclusions can be drawn now:
1. The effect of homeopathic potencies on healthy plants is generally minimal (2–3% max.) but statistically well-supported.
2. Using homeopathic potencies on stressed or sick plants can produce a stronger reaction (up to 20%).
3. Some trials have shown evidence of an effect of ultra-highly diluted homeopathic potencies (which are not in line with the classical pharmacological view).
4. There is multiple evidence that homeopathic potencies have a regulatory or balancing effect; it has been observed, for instance, that under the influence of potentized homeopathic substances the developmental variability of plants is generally lower.

These results support, if only indirectly, the following two fundamental tenets of homeopathy:
1. The action of homeopathic potencies is primarily regulatory and can therefore be more easily observed in the sick than in the healthy organism.
2. Substances can also induce specific reactions in living organisms if they are highly diluted (potentized).

4.2.3 Animal studies

Poisoning studies are a common and well-reproduced standard model. They go back to research done by Lapp and Wurmser in the 1950s and are based on the following premise: test animals are poisoned with toxic substances and then protected or detoxified with homeopathic potencies of the same poison. The breaking-down rate of the poison in urine and faeces is accelerated. Among the best-controlled blind trials are still those on arsenic poisoning conducted by Cazin and Gaborit in the 1980s. The same model is used for the artificial induction of diseases in animals, for example, the use of potentized alloxan to protect animals from diabetes mellitus induced by alloxan poisoning. A meta-analysis (Linde et al. 1994) of 105 intoxication trials showed clear, clinically relevant and significantly positive effects for homeopathic treatment.

Bastide's research team demonstrated in their investigations that high homeopathic potencies of hormones can fully replace the material hormone deficiency in chickens (Bastide et al. 1983, Youbicier-Simo et al. 1996). Endler's team arrived at similar results: highly-potentized homeopathic thyroxin slows down the development of amphibians (frogs); however, the effect was restricted to animals with (artificially or naturally) raised hormone levels (Endler et al. 2003, Zausner et al. 2002).

These studies also support the proposition that homeopathic potencies have primarily a regulatory effect, i.e. they restore balance to destabilized organisms.

4.2.4 In vitro studies with human cells

The most proven in-vitro model involving human research material is the human basophil degranulation test (HBDT) known from allergology. It is based on the fact that in allergic reactions the basophil granulocytes degranulate after exposure to an allergen. In countless trials with several variations it was possible to supply significant, multiply reproduced evidence that the BDT was influenced by high homeopathic potencies of histamines, bee poison and other substances capable of inducing allergic reactions (Belon et al. 2004).

4.2.5 Conclusion: fundamental preclinical research

The tenet of homeopathy that very high dilutions of medicinal substances (homeopathic potencies) are able to induce specific effects in living organisms is supported by quite a large number of high-quality trials in fundamental preclinical research. Homeopathic remedies, moreover, seem to have a regulatory, i.e. balancing or normalising, effect and possess a specific physical structure. Fundamental preclinical research is unable to supply statements regarding the other mainstays of homeopathy: the simile principle and drug proving on the healthy subject (non-transferability).

4.3 Clinical trials

4.3.1 Classification

The historical evidence arising from widespread clinical use of homeopathy in the 19th and 20th centuries must not be excluded from our discussion of modern research methods (Kaufmann 1971; 20th-century research has as yet not been fully evaluated).

Homeopathy trials can be classified according to content or chronology (based on Dean 2004, p. 96):
1. Observational studies of classical homeopathy for various indications on individual cases and small collectives (1821–1835)
2. Open comparative studies of classical homeopathy with conventional, expectant (non-) therapy or with, partly unintentional, placebo treatment (1830–1890)
3. Controlled studies of nosological clinical homeopathy (1914–1953)
4. Randomized clinical studies of isopathy and classical, clinical and complex homeopathy (1950–2004 and beyond)
5. Epidemiological studies (1990-2004 and beyond)

The large 19th-century studies (items 1 and 2) involving participant numbers that have never again been reached since then have so far been rarely assessed for clinical efficacy (e.g. Leary 1994).

Most 20th-century clinical homeopathy studies (75–90%) available today (items 3 and 4) tested isopathy and clinical and complex homeopathy (Dean 2004, p. 212), and there are severe restrictions to their reproducibility in the Swiss practice (cf. Sect. 4.1 Introduction and research problems).

Next to drug provings, observational studies are the main form of system-immanent research in homeopathy. Prospective and retrospective observations of selected collectives are preferred to the 'gold standard' of conventional clinical research (prospective randomized clinical double-blind trials) as the former possess higher external validity and significance for homeopathy.

Randomized controlled trials (RCT) are diametrically opposed to the homeopathic method. In contrast to conventional pharmacotherapy, homeopathy knows only one definite verum in the individual case. It is not the homeopathic remedy as pharmacological substance as such that is effective. It becomes effective only when it was chosen to exactly suit the individuality of the patient in question (hypothesis) and when its action on the patient's symptoms has been confirmed (verification). Placebo control certainly presents a problem for clinical research into homeotherapy and, as a rule, it reduces a study's internal and external validity. Because of the meticulous case-taking and close interaction between physician and patient, the value attached to individual symptoms, and the self-observation necessary for the selection and repeated application of a substance, one soon loses track of individual reactions and durations of drug effects in all but the simplest cases if it is not clear whether verum or placebo was used (Mattmann-Allamand 1998).

More recent epidemiological studies evaluate the whole system of 'classical homeopathic therapy' under 'real-world conditions', which allows them to draw conclusions regarding individual and collective effectiveness (Becker-Witt et al. 2003, 2004; Güthlin et al. 2004).

The inclusion of the characteristic properties of both research systems in mutually acceptable protocols certainly requires a sophisticated methodology.

4.3.2 An outline of clinical trials

a) Clinical trials in selected areas:
   Dean (2004) categorizes the evidence gained in homeopathy studies up to 1998 according to the various homeopathic methods. Indications regarding clinical efficacy can be found in a survey by Mathie (2003) for the following conditions: diarrhoea in children, fibromyalgia, hay fever, influenza-like infections, (various) pains, side effects of radio- and chemotherapy, sprains, and infections of the upper respiratory tract. The WHO study (in preparation) adds otitis media as a ninth diagnosis.
   Further indications of positive evidence are found for the following diagnoses/indications (adapted from Righetti 1988 and 1999, Wein 2002, Dean 2004 and Mathie 2003):
   - mustard gas poisoning (Paterson 1943)
   - diphtheria epidemics (Paterson and Boyd 1941, Hess 1942, Schmitz 1942, Schwartzhaupt 1942, Schoeler 1948, Dean 2004)
   - acute pharyngitis (Fournier 1979, Bauhof 1982, Frei 2000)
   - otitis media (Jacobs et al. 2001; Frei and Thurneysen 2001)

— traumatology (dentistry: Ives 1984, Albertini et al. 1984, Michaud 1981)
— obstetrics (Arnal-Lasserre 1987, Hochstrasser 1999, Hochstrasser and Mattmann 1999)
— asthma (Boucinhas and de Medeiros Boucinhas 1990, Freitas et al. 1995, Reilly et al. 1994, Lara-Marquez et al. 1997, Matusiewicz et al. 1995, 1997 and 1999, Riveron-Garrote et al. 1998).

This summary of evidence of clinical efficacy gleaned from homeopathy research is not complete, as the 'old' literature has been processed to only a limited extent (Dean 2004) and the existent 'overall surveys' (such as Clausius 1998) were carried out only selectively.

b) Large-scale observational studies / outcome studies:
A number of recent, mostly practice-oriented, observational studies are based on individual diagnoses or diagnosis groups and verify positive effects in favour of homeopathy (e.g. Hochstrasser and Mattmann 1999; Strosser & Weiser 2000; Heger et al. 2000 and Riley et al. 2001; IIPCOS-1/-2; Muscari-Tomaioli et al. 2001; Dias Brunini 2002; Thompson and Reilly 2003).

More recent longitudinal epidemiological studies have been carried out under real practice conditions involving quite high patient numbers and broad diagnosis groups. Especially in Germany and also in Switzerland, they have shown clearly positive results (e.g. Becker-Witt et al. 2003 and 2004, Güthlin et al. 2003, also results from PEK component II). The two latter trials include control groups.

c) Meta-analyses and (systematic) reviews:
Meta-analyses and reviews of predominantly conventional trials also indicate efficacy. They are dealt with in more detail in Chap. 9.

4.3.3 Future research

A systematic worldwide review of the literature on homeopathic trials which takes into account historical evidence, retrospective studies and single case reports and consults homeopathy experts will be necessary as a basis for further clinical research. Homeopathy requires adequate and more comprehensive research structures in the future. It should then, through single case and cohort studies, identify the aspects that can be addressed by way of controlled clinical investigation. Aspects that are inherent in homeopathy (theory, methods and treatment outcomes) should also be worked on.

What research methods can do justice to the homeopathic approach (external validity) as well as to its claims for outside recognition (internal validity)?

— The method that is best suited to prove homeopathic effectiveness in the clinical situation on the basis of individual remedy selection is the single-case observation (intraindividual approach) on many patients and on cases of chronic disease over a sufficiently long follow-up period. Although numerous single case reports have been published, a great number of case histories are still awaiting evaluation in homeopathic practices.

— Large systematic observational studies (outcome studies) are carried out under real practice conditions, thus meeting the validity requirements of both homeopathy and evidence-based medicine. If at all possible they should include control groups.

— Randomized controlled trials (RCTs) with individual prescription are very complex and difficult to carry out, especially in chronic cases, and therefore ethically questionable for both sides.

— The only exception, if any, is represented by randomized controlled trials with narrowly defined symptom groups or reactions where one standard treatment covers the majority of cases, as in traumatology. Difficulties can still arise here with regard to the homogeneity and recruitment of the groups and the lack of individualisation.

- Through 'matching', individual homeopathic treatment can be compared with treatment in a conventional medical control group.
- Comparison of the systems as such: homeopathic versus conventional general practice treatment with a sufficiently high number of patients over a sufficiently long period of time (cf. Mattmann-Allamand 1998 and Mattmann-Allamand, personal information: suggestion of cohort study, Schweizerischer Nationalfonds SNF 2005; suggestion homeopathy study on PEK component IV, 2001; application NRP 34, 1992).

4.3.4 Summary clinical studies

Since its inception over 200 years ago, homeopathy has been based on empirical research. Apart from this system-immanent research, homeopathy has so far lacked a tradition of systematic research. Barring a few exceptions, homeopathy has existed mostly outside the universities in the recent past. In contrast to mainstream medicine, the practice of homeopathy gains little from conventional trials. There is no interested pharmaceutical industry nor are there potent sponsors; research infrastructures and appropriate research concepts are also lacking. The physicians are individual practitioners who show little interest in this kind of research; even experienced qualified homeopaths are unaware of the outcomes of such 'irrelevant' trials.

The past decades have seen a rising number of experimental and clinical investigations based on the approach of conventional medicine. The standard methods applied in recent years are so incompatible with the homeopathic approach that a qualified comparison of systems remains impossible if there is no adaptation and integration of homeopathic methods. Because such studies have hardly anything in common with homeopathic practice – a fact that considerably reduces their external and model validity – they increase the likelihood of false-negative results. Here too, the absence of the evidence of effectiveness ('negative study outcomes') is certainly not evidence of ineffectiveness.

In spite of these difficulties, there are many trials that demonstrate the experimental effect and clinical efficacy of homeopathic methods also by conventional medical standards (cf. Chaps. 9 and 10).

Homeopathy will need appropriate research opportunities and structures in the future. Epidemiological studies should be designed to allow for a genuine system comparison between conventional and homeopathic approaches without distorting the homeopathic method. They should integrate specific research approaches of both disciplines without excluding any of their essential aspects. This is best achieved by means of observational practice studies conducted with higher numbers of patients over a sufficiently long period of time. In addition, promising and meaningful experimental and clinical studies could be carried out and replicated under consideration of homeopathic principles to provide evidence of its basic effectiveness.

4.4 References

Albertini H, Goldberg W, Sanguy BB, Toulza C (1985) Homeopathic treatment of dental neuralgia using arnica and hypericum: a summary of 60 observations. J Am Inst Homeopathy 8:126–128
Arnal-Laserre MN (1987) Préparation à l'accouchement par homéopathie: expérimentation en double insu versus placebo. Dissertation, Academie de Paris Université René Descartes, Paris

Bastide M, Doucet-Jaboeuf M, Daurat V (1983) Action immunopharmacologique des préparations de thymus et d'hormone thymique utilisées à doses infinitésimales. Homeopathie Française 71:185–189

Bauhof G (1982) Die homöopathische Behandlung der Angina. Dissertation, Freiburg i Br.

Baumgartner S, Heusser P, Thurneysen A (1998) Methodological standards and problems in preclinical homeopathic potency research. Forschende Komplementärmedizin und Klassische Naturheilkunde 5:27–32

Baumgartner S, Shah D, Heusser P, Thurneysen A (2000) Homeopathic dilutions: is there a potential for applications in organic plant production? In: Aföldi T, Lockeretz W, Niggli U (eds) IFOAM 2000 – The world grows organic. vdf Hochschulverlag, Zurich, pp 97–100

Becker-Witt C, Weisshuhn TER, Lüdtke R, Willich SN (2003) Quality assessment of physical research in homeopathy. J Altern Complement Med 9:113–132

Becker-Witt C, Lüdtke R, Weisshuhn TER, Willich SN (2004) Diagnoses and treatment in homeopathic medical practice. Forschende Komplementärmedizin und Klassische Naturheilkunde 11:98-103

Belon P, Cumps J, Ennis M, Mannaioni PF, Roberfroid M, Sainte-Laudy J, Wiegant FA (2004) Histamine dilutions modulate basophil activation. Inflamm Res 53:181–188

Betti L, Borghini F, Nani D (2003) Plant models for fundamental research in homeopathy. Homeopathy 92:129–130

Boissel JP, Cucherat M, Haugh M, Gauthier E (1996) Critical literature review on the effectiveness of homeopathy: overview of data from homeopathic medicine trials. In: Homeopathic Medicine Research Group. Report to the Commission of the European Union Communities. pp 196–210

Boucinhas JC, de Medeiros Boucinhas ID (1990) Prophylaxie des crises d'asthme bronchique chez l'enfant par l'usage de Poumon histamine 5CH. Homeopathie Française 78:35–39

Brigo B, Serpelloni G (1991) Homeopathic treatment of migraines: a randomized double-blind controlled study of 60 cases. Berl J Res Homeopathy 1:98–106

Cazin JC, Gaborit JL (1983) Etude pharmacologique de la rétention et de la mobilisation de l'arsenic. In: Boiron J, Abecassis J et al (eds) Aspects de la recherche en homeopathie, vol I. Boiron, Sainte-Foy-lès-Lyon

Clausius N (1998) Kontrollierte klinische Studien zur Homöopathie – eine systematische Übersichtsarbeit mit Metaanalyse. KVC-Verlag, Essen

Cucherat M, Haugh MC, Gooch M, Boissel JP (2000) Evidence of clinical efficacy of homeopathy. A meta-analysis of clinical trials. Homeopathic Medicines Research Advisory Group (HMRAG). Eur J Clin Pharmacol 56:27–33

Dean ME (2004) The Trials of homeopathy – origins, structure and development. KVC-Verlag, Essen

Demangeat JL, Gries P, Poitevin B, Droesbeke JJ, Zahaf T, Maton F, Piérart C, Muller RN (2004) Low-field NMR water proton longitudinal relaxation in ultra-highly diluted aqueous solutions of silica-lactose prepared in glass material for pharmaceutical use. Appl Magn Reson 26:465–481

Dias Brunini CR (2002) Qualidade de vida e abordagem homeopatica em criança asmaticas. (Quality of life and homeopathic approach in asthmatic children.) Infanto 10:18–21

Elia V, Niccoli M (2000) New physico-chemical properties of water induced by mechanical treatments. A calorimetric study at 25°C. J Thermal Analysis Calorimetry 61:527–537

Endler PC, Lüdtke R, Heckmann C, Zausner C, Lassnig H, Scherer-Pongratz W, Haidvogl M, Frass M (2003) Pretreatment with thyroxine (10-(8) parts by weight) enhances a 'curative' effect of homeopathically prepared thyroxine (10-(13)) on lowland frogs. Forschende Komplementärmedizin und Klassische Naturheilkunde 10:137–142

Fournier H (1979) Traitements homéopathiques des angines. Dissertation, Nantes

Frei H (2000) Homöopathische Behandlung der Tonsillopharyngitiden bei Kindern. Schweiz Z GanzheitsMed 12:37–40

Frei H, Thurneysen A (2001) Treatment for hyperactive children: homeopathy and methylphenidate compared in a family setting. Br Homeopathic J 90:183–188

Freitas LAS de, Goldenstein E, Sanna OM (1995) A relação médico–paciente indireta e o tratmento homeopático na asma infantil. Rev Homeopatia – APH (Sao Paulo) 60:26–31

Gerhard I, Reimers G, Keller C, Schmück M (1993) Vergleich homöopathischer Einzelmittel mit konventioneller Hormontherapie. Therapeutikon 7:309–315

Güthlin C, Lange O, Walach H (2004) Measuring the effects of acupuncture and homeopathy in general practice: an uncontrolled prospective documentation approach. BMC Public Health 4:6

Heger M, Riley DS, Haidvogl M (2000) International integrative primary care outcomes study (IIPCOS-2): an international research project of homeopathy in primary care. Br Homeopathic J 89 [Suppl 1]:S10–13

Hess FO (1942) Nützt uns die Homöopathie bei der Diphtherie-Behandlung? Munch Med Wochenschr 13:296

Hochstrasser B (1999) Lebensqualität von schwangeren Frauen in Abhängigkeit von einer homöopathischen oder schulmedizinischen Betreuungsform und vom Schwangerschaftsverlauf. Forschende Komplementärmedizin 6 [Suppl 1]:23–25

Hochstrasser B, Mattmann P (1999) Mainstream medicine versus complementary medicine (homeopathic) interven-
tion: a critical methodology study of care in pregnancy. Forschende Komplementärmedizin 6 [Suppl 1]: 20–22
Ives G (1984) A double-blind pilot study of Arnica in dental extraction. Midlands Homeopathic Research Group.
Communications 11:71–74
Jacobs J, Springer DA, Crothers D (2001) Homeopathic treatment of acute otitis media in children: A preliminary
randomized placebo-controlled trial. Pediatric Infectious Dis J 20:177–183
Kaufmann M (1971) Homeopathy in America, the rise and fall of a medical heresy. Johns Hopkins University Press,
Baltimore
Kleijnen J, Knipschild P, ter Riet G (1991) Clinical trials of homeopathy. BMJ 302:316–323
Lapp C, Wurmser L (1955) Mobilisation de l'arsenic fixé chez le cobaye sous l'influence de doses infinitésimales
d'arséniate de sodium. Therapie 10:625–638
Lapp C, Wurmser L, Kautrelle J (1958) Mobilisation du bismuth fixé chez le cobaye sous l'influence de doses infi-
nitésimales d'un sel de bismuth. Therapie 13:438–450
Lara-Marquez ML, Pocino M, Rodriguez F, Carvallo GE, Ortega CF, Rodruguez C (1997) Homeopathic treatment for
atopic asthma lung function and immunological outcomes in a randomized clinical trial in Venzuela. Proc
52nd Congress of the Liga Medicorum Homeopathia Internationalis. Seattle, Washington, USA, p 73
Leary B (1994) Cholera 1854 (update). Br Homeopathic J 83:117–121
Linde K, Jonas WB, Melchart D, Worku F, Wagner H, Eitel F (1994) Critical review and meta-analysis of serial agi-
tated dilutions. Hum Exp Toxicol 13:481–492
Linde K, Clausius N, Ramirez G, Melchart D, Eitel F, Hedges LV, Jonas WB (1997) Are the effects of homeopathy
placebo effects? A meta-analysis of randomized, placebo controlled trials. Lancet 350:834–843
Linde K, Melchart D (1998) Randomized controlled trials of individual homeopathy: a state-of-the-art review.
J Altern Complement Med 4:371–388
Mathie RT (2003) The research evidence base for homeopathy: a fresh assessment of the literature. Homeopathy
92:84–91
Mattmann-Allamand P (1998) Indirekter Wirksamkeitsnachweis durch den Vergleich ganzer Therapiesysteme
ohne Placebo-Gruppen. Hoffnung für die homöopathische Wirksamkeitsforschung? Forschende Komplemen-
tärmedizin 5 [Suppl 1]:131–135
Matusiewicz R (1995) Wirksamkeit von Engystol N bei Bronchialasthma und kortikoidabhängiger Therapie. Biol
Med 24:242–246
Matusiewicz R (1997) The homeopathic treatment of corticosteroid-dependent asthma. A double-blind, placebo-
controlled study. Biomed Ther 15:117–122
Matusiewicz R, Wasniewski J, Sterna-Bazanska A, Hülsberg M (1999) Behandlung des chronischen Asthma bron-
chiale mit einem homöopathischen Komplexmittel. Erfahrungsheilkunde 48:367–372
Muscari-Tomaioli G, Allegri R, Miali E, Pomposelli R. Tubia P, Targhetta A, Castellini M, Bellavite P (2001) Observa-
tional study of quality of life in patients with headache, receiving homeopathic treatment. Br Homeopathic
J 90:189–197
Michaud J (1981) Action d'Apis mel. et d'Arnica dans la prévention des oedèmes post-opératoires en chirurgie
maxilo-faciale. Dissertation, Nantes
Paterson J (1944) Report on mustard gas experiments (Glasgow and London). J Am Inst Homeopathy 37:47–50,
88–92
Paterson J, Boyd WE (1941) Potency action. A preliminary study of the alteration of the Schick-test by a homeo-
pathic potency. Br Homeopathic J 31:301–309
Poitevin B (1987) Le Devenir de l'Homéopathie - Eléments de théorie et de recherche. Doin Editeurs, Paris
Reilly D, Taylor M (1986) Is homeopathy a placebo response? Lancet 2:881–886
Reilly D, Taylor MA, Beattie NG, Campbell JH, McSharry C, Aitchison TC (1994) Is evidence for homeopathy repro-
ducible? Lancet 344:1601–1606
Righetti M (1988) Forschung in der Homöopathie. Burgdorf, Göttingen
Righetti M Homöopathie: Grundlagen, Anwendungsgebiete und mögliche Ansätze zu Forschungsstudien. 1999.
Available at: - HYPERLINK http://www.homeodoctor.ch/Righetti.htm
Riley D, Fischer M, Singh B, Haidvogl M, Heger M (2001) Homeopathy and conventional medicine: an outcome
study comparing effectiveness in a primary care setting. J Altern Complement Med 7:149–159
Riveron-Garrote M, Fernandez-Argüelles R, Morón-Rodriguez F, Campistrou-Labaut, JL (1998) Ensayo clínico con-
trolado aleatorizado del tratamiento homeopático del asma bronquial. Bol Mexicano Homeopatía 31:54–61
Schoeler H (1948) Über die wissenschaftlichen Grundlagen der Homöopathie. Professorial dissertation, Faculty
of Medicine at the University of Leipzig

Schmitz 1942, quoted from Righetti M (1988) Forschung in der Homöopathie. Burgdorf, Göttingen

Schwartzhaupt 1942, quoted from Righetti M (1988) Forschung in der Homöopathie. Burgdorf, Göttingen

Strosser W, Weiser M (2000) Lebensqualität bei Patienten mit Schwindel – Homöopathikum im Doppelblind-Vergleich. Biol Med 29:242–247

Thompson EA, Reilly D (2003) The homeopathic approach to the treatment of symptoms of oestrogen withdrawal in breast cancer patients. A prospective observational study. Homeopathy 92:131–134

Vickers AJ (1999) Independent replication of pre-clinical research in homeopathy: a systematic review. Forschende Komplementärmedizin und Klassische Naturheilkunde 6:311–320

Walach H (1986) Homöopathie als Basistherapie. Haug, Heidelberg

Walach H, Haeusler W, Lowes T, Mussbach D, Schamell U, Springer W, Stritzl G, Gaus W, Haag G (1997) Classical homeopathic treatment of chronic headaches. Cephalalgia 17:11–18

Wein C (2002) Qualitätsaspekte klinischer Studien zur Homöopathie. KVC-Verlag, Essen

Weingärtner O (1992) Homöopathische Potenzen. Springer-Verlag, Berlin, Heidelberg, New York

Weingärtner O (2002) Kernresonanz-Spektroskopie in der Homöopathieforschung. KVC-Verlag, Essen

Whitmarsh TE, Coleston-Shields DM, Steiner DJ (1997) Double blind, randomized, placebo-controlled study of homeopathic prophylaxis of migraine. Cephalalgia 17:600–604

Wiesenauer M, Gaus W, Bohnacker U, Häussler S (1989) Wirksamkeitsprüfung von homöopathischen Kombinationspräparaten bei Sinusitis. Ergebnisse einer randomisierten Doppelblindstudie unter Praxisbedingungen. Arzneimittelforschung 39:620–625

Wiesenauer M, Gaus W (1991) Wirksamkeitsnachweis eines Homöopathikums bei chronischer Polyarthritis. Eine randomisierte Doppelblindstudie bei niedergelassenen Ärzten. Aktuelle Rheumatol 16:1–9

Wolter H (1980) Wirksamkeitsnachweis von Caulophyllum D 30 bei der Wehenschwäche des Schweines im doppelten Blindversuch. In: Gebhardt KH (ed) Beweisbare Homöopathie. Haug, Heidelberg

Youbicier-Simo BJ, Boudard F, Mékaouche M, Baylé JD, Bastide M (1996) A role for bursa fabricii and bursin in the ontogeny of the pineal biosynthetic activity in the chicken. J Pineal Res 21:35–43

Zausner C, Lassnig H, Endler PC, Scherer-Pongratz W, Haidvogl M, Frass M, Kastberger G, Lüdtke R (2002) Die Wirkung von 'homöopathisch' zubereitetem Thyroxin auf die Metamorphose von Hochlandamphibien – Ergebnisse einer multizentrischen Kontrollstudie. Perfusion. 15:268–276

General problems with clinical trials in research

Peter F. Matthiessen, Gudrun Bornhöft

5.1   The Problems with Randomized Clinical Trials

Evidence-based medicine (EBM) has as its aim and concern the identification and evaluation of the entire body of published evidence concerning a medical problem with a view to making the results available, assessable and easily usable in medical practice. It therefore sees itself first and foremost as an instrument of medical decision-making with the task of supporting physicians in their day-to-day work with patients. EBM's central stipulation is the provision of external evidence in the form of scientifically verified knowledge.

Following a scientific majority decision, the following classification into four levels of evidence[1] was agreed upon:

Ia: evidence obtained from meta-analysis of randomized controlled trials
Ib: evidence obtained from at least one randomized controlled trial
IIa: evidence obtained from at least one controlled trial without randomisation
IIb: evidence obtained from at least one quasi-experimental study
III: evidence obtained from non-experimental, descriptive studies
IV: evidence obtained from expert committee reports/opinions, consensus conferences and/or clinical experience of respected authorities.

Although Sackett et al. (1997), as co-initiators of EBM, envisaged a synthesis of external evidence and individual professional expertise ('EBM … never replaces clinical skills, clinical judgement and clinical experience') it has become customary in EBM to accept as 'evidence' only the results obtained by means of formalized data generation, evaluation and presentation procedures. Sackett had pointed out that EBM was not limited to randomized trials and meta-analyses, but in the wake of the ensuing EBM euphoria it has become established practice to rely solely on the results of randomized controlled clinical trials (RCTs) and their meta-analyses. At the same time it is becoming increasingly apparent that EBM, while serving a valuable instrumental purpose, has its own inherent shortcomings, like any other scientific method, which can give rise to system-immanent distortions and a systematic error potential once the methodical tool has become independent and claims universal validity. This also applies to the one-sided, if not exclusive, reliance on the results of (preferably double-blinded) controlled randomized trials (RCTs) as the 'gold standard' in supplying evidence of effectiveness.

The circumstances described below (cf. also Matthiessen 2003, 2005) are often ignored by the scientific community as well as in the decision-making processes of the various health care systems, despite the fact that they have become the centre of much discussion (not only in complementary but also in conventional medicine):

1. The absence of a positive or any RCT result is no proof of ineffectiveness ('absence of evidence is not evidence of absence', Altman and Bland 1995); there is a danger that effective therapies are eliminated because there is no RCT proof of their efficacy.
2. A negative RCT result is also not valid proof of ineffectiveness because many factors can be involved in causing false-negative RCT results. Vice versa, the absence of many factors that are excluded by the RCT design can be responsible for false-negative results, such as a disturbed doctor-patient relationship, non-compliance, drop-outs (with ITT analysis), complementary and compensatory therapy, but also mega-studies with their – necessarily – simplified study design.

1   EBM evidence grading by AHCPR (Agency for Health Care Policy and Research) 1992. Cf. also SIGN 50 (2004); for assignation of grades cf. p 33.

3. Individualized medical care is more and more being replaced by standardized treatment methods to ensure comparability and reproducibility of study outcomes.
4. Trial results can be significantly positive even though only a small percentage of patients experience genuine benefit from the trial. This applies particularly to trials with large, but generally heterogeneous, patient collectives. The results do not allow for conclusions as to which patients (or subgroups) benefited and which did not benefit (or sustained damage from the treatment). In preventive medicine, a 'number needed to treat' (NNT) of 100–200 subjects is still considered sensible! One must ask how many people can be expected to use a medication that is of no benefit to them in order to help one individual in the group. Study results can, on the other hand, come out negative although a percentage of the patients drew definite benefit from the treatment. With most trials the statistical significance is not enough to discriminate between even major differences in the subgroups (cf. Niroomand 2004).
5. Reproducibility is surprisingly low even with 'hard' RCTs (rigorous inclusion criteria, end points with minimal subjectivity). There are also ethical concerns which prohibit repetition of RCTs with a positive outcome (in favour of the test intervention) because the patients in the control group would be denied a treatment that is known to be effective.
6. This is not the only ethical reason why there needs to be genuine openness ('equipoise') at the beginning of a randomized trial, i.e. neither physician nor patient have a preference regarding a particular treatment. The fact that a patient has given his or her 'informed consent' does not avoid the problem, since the responsibility cannot simply be placed on the patient, certainly not according to the Declaration of the World Medical Association: 'The responsibility for the human subject must always rest with a medically qualified person and never rest on the subject of the research, even though the subject has given consent.' (Quoted from Kienle et al. 2006b). Equipoise, in fact, applies only to the classical usage of RCTs, i.e. the testing of new medicines on which the terms 'preclinical' and 'clinical research' and 'phase I, II, III and IV trials' are based. It is doubtful whether RCTs are suitable for the evaluation of complex therapeutic procedures or of entire therapy systems that have been part of the day-to-day primary health care provision for decades.
7. In view of the ethical problems mentioned, it appears doubtful whether the authorities have the right to insist on randomized trials, i.e. evidence of inferior treatment and discrimination of control group patients, as a basis for decisions concerning health service reimbursement. To quote Gerhard Kienle: 'If authorities, beyond the ethically and legally demanded duty of self-sacrifice, make *experiments on humans* a precondition for the availability of certain medicines to the physician, necessary to fulfil his treatment obligation, then they are exerting a compulsion through which the study participant will become the means to an end. This act falls within Kant's definition of immorality.' (Kienle 1974, p 23, quoted from Kienle et al. 2006b).
8. 'Recently the discussion for and against mammography screening exemplified how different professional evidence-based reviews of identical clinical studies could nevertheless arrive at different conclusions and even opposing recommendations on treatment' (cf. Dickersin 2003, quoted from Kienle et al. 2006b). Not only the RCT results but also the results obtained from systematic reviews of RCTs can show considerable divergence.
9. The thematic orientation of RCTs is often not relevant to problems of health care or the needs of patients, but is driven by subjective interests (career, sponsors). Due to the enormous costs involved, clinical research has become the domain of the pharmaceutical industry and is governed primarily by licensing and marketing interests. The generation of evidence for treatments that promise success but not financial profit or for non-pharmacological therapies is therefore considered dispensable.

The Swiss Federal Social Insurance Office's (FSIO[2]) *Manual for the standardisation of clinical and economic evaluation of medical technologies*[3], on which our assessment is also based, explicitly mentions as appropriate test methods those which

a) Evaluate the treatment method under consideration in its entirety
b) Take into proper consideration the realistic research possibilities in practice
c) Permit inference to the target population that is being treated in practice

Based on these requirements, and contrary to the usual evidence grading, evaluation methods that involve no experimental change in the medical intervention (such as case studies) are considered preferable, as they are better able to reflect the health care reality.

In this reality, the autonomous patients of today express clear preferences concerning the physicians they consult and the treatment or therapy they favour, and they reject randomisation. This at least emerged from all the – attempted – comparative studies within our UMR/UMK[4]-Methoden project coordination (1986–1996). Comparisons between conventional and complementary medical therapies can therefore in principle hardly be randomized.

Patients who – after having been fully informed – agree to randomisation usually belong to a highly selected population whose real-world representativeness is doubtful.

Misleading accounts claim that a high percentage (80%) of today's mainstream medicine is based on EBM (Ernst 2004). The literature quoted (Gill et al. 1996) suggests a different situation: although 82 of 122 consecutive patient treatments in general practice were 'evidence-based', only 31 (a quarter) were supported by randomized trials. The remaining 51 'evidence-based' therapeutic measures relied on 'convincing non-experimental evidence'. The authors therefore demanded 'an appropriate paradigm of evidence-based practice rather than that determined solely by clinical trials' (Gill et al. 1996). 'We believe that for general practice, and possibly in other settings too, the most important evidence may be found in developing alternative methodologies which complement conclusions from randomized controlled trials' (Gill et al. 1996). 'These statements do not support an EBM-foundation of primary care, but rather stress the importance of the evidence generated by clinical judgment and experience, and of the need for a methodology that can adequately cover this type of evidence' (quoted from Kienle et al. 2006b).

Heusser (2001) illustrated the extent to which other methods solve the problem of transferring 'biased' study results to real-world practice or generate new problems (◘ Table 5.1).

We therefore consider the following tacit assumptions in the usage and interpretation of RCTS to be questionable or false:

- The treatment reality can be adapted to the RCT model and thus allow for an assessment that corresponds to the model.
- The RCT result can be projected back to the treatment reality and is valid there (external validity).
- A formally correct RCT is equally safe from false-positive and false-negative results (neutral test validity).

In our evaluation of the studies analysed in the present HTA we decided against grading the study types and merely described the EBM evidence level in the data synthesis.

---

2   BSV Bundesverband für Sozialversicherung
3   Handbuch zur Standardisierung der medizinischen und wirtschaftlichen Bewertung medizinischer Leistungen
4   UMK unkonventionelle Methoden der Krebsbekämpfung; UMR unkonventionelle medizinische Richtungen – non-conventional medical approaches UMK unkonventionelle Krebsbekämpfung – non-conventional cancer therapies

◘ **Table 5.1** Comparison: the advantages and disadvantages of various methods of gaining medical knowledge (Heusser 2001)

Method	Gain/advantage	Loss/disadvantage
1. clinical experience	overview over real practice situation incl. subjective and objective, qualitative and quantitative individual factors	documentation often insufficient; information not precise; problems of remembering
2. case reports retrospective	real practice situation documented, still including subjective and objective, qualitative and quantitative individual factors	documentation often incomplete; case selection
3. retrospective study	real practice situation; quantitative evaluation of all patient files	documentation often incomplete; limited to quantitative data
4. prospective observational study	real practice situation; complete documentation; possibility of retaining subjective and qualitative factors	spontaneity of medical decision impaired
5. one-arm prospective study	experiment; uniform therapy, 'objectivity': independent of treating physician	impairment of medical competence, individualisation and flexibility of treatment
6. controlled trial	systematic comparability	impairment of medical competence; sub-optimal treatment in control groups
7. randomized trial	optimal comparability of patient groups	impairment of doctor-patient relationship; loss of medical competence
8. double-blind trial	equal chance for subjective expectations, treatment and observation; 'objective' treatment	loss of relationship between doctor-patient-medication and loss of context

The terms 'quasi-experimental study', 'cohort study', 'clinical observational study', 'outcome study' etc. are not always used uniformly. If it was apparent from the documentation, we assigned evidence level IIb to studies with a contemporary comparable control group ('quasi-parallel group design'), and evidence level III to studies with no or insufficient control (e.g. historical comparison only or retrospective evaluation). Differentiation between evidence levels IIa and IIb was dependent on whether the choice/allocation of treatment took place within the trial setting (IIa) or whether data from a 'natural' treatment course were evaluated (IIb). Case reports were assigned evidence level IV, but a more differentiated distinction between anecdotal and well-documented single-case descriptions would be desirable in future.

5.2 The Risk of Bias in Clinical Trials

Instead of just formally evaluating the studies, we examined their content for bias. Wherever this was possible on the basis of the data available we searched for bias due to methodical deficiencies (internal validity) or whether the studies were not or only partially transferable to our research because they inadequately reflected the real health care situation.

- ■ **Terminology:**

Internal validity (IV) refers to the methodological quality of a study, or more precisely, 'the confidence that the trial design, conduct and analysis has minimized or avoided biases in its treatment comparison' (Moher et al. 1999). It is seen as 'a measure of the strength of the association between exposure or intervention and outcome within a study', SIGN 2002).

The term *external validity (EV)* is not always used in the same sense. It can be synonymous with 'generalisability, relevance and transferability: the degree to which the results of an observation hold true in other settings' (Alderson et al. 2004); or it can refer to 'the extent to which the effects observed in a study are applicable outside of the study – in routine practice', (Khan et al. 2001). In general it describes the transferability to possible target groups ('[whether] the effects observed in a study truly reflect what can be expected in a target population beyond the people included in the study', [Alderson et al. 2004]), target settings or individual patients in the context of a treatment decision.

The term *model validity (MV)* is not generally known in medical circles. It describes the conformity between the study setting and an ideal procedure ('state of the art' of the intervention under consideration, e.g. classical homeopathy) with regard to indication, intervention, expertise of the therapist etc. (cf. Wein 2002).

The terms 'internal and external validity' are of methodological origin (internal validity: the methodical quality of a study; external validity: its value for the treating physician, for instance). They must not be confused with the terms *internal and external evidence* (cf. Kienle 2001), which describe the point of view of the physician: 'internal evidence' is the reference value for a treatment decision derived from the physician's knowledge and experience (a factor which is systematically eliminated or at least minimized in RCTs!); external evidence denotes the evidence generated independently of the physician (e.g. in clinical studies).

In the present HTA internal and external validity were determined. Both validity assessments were described separately while the systematic evaluation of the bias factors known to influence internal validity – selection, performance, attrition and detection bias – was also applied to the external validity.

- ■ **Terminology:**

Bias (distortion) is defined in the Cochrane Collaboration Handbook (Alderson et al. 2004) as 'a systematic error or deviation in results or inferences. In studies of the effects of healthcare, bias can arise from systematic differences in the groups that are compared (selection bias), the care that is provided, or exposure to other factors apart from the intervention of interest (performance bias), withdrawals or exclusions of people entered into the study (attrition bias) or how outcomes are assessed (detection bias)' (see ◻ Fig. 5.1).

The literature includes more factors and variations (Sackett 1979, Kienle 2005), but the present HTA evaluates the main categories only.

The terms established for the internal validity of RCTs that refer to the comparison between a verum and a control group within one trial setting were analogized to determine external validity, i.e. for the comparison between the study group and a target population (patients who use a complementary medical therapy such as homeopathy in Switzerland). ◻ Table 5.2 illustrates this analogisation.

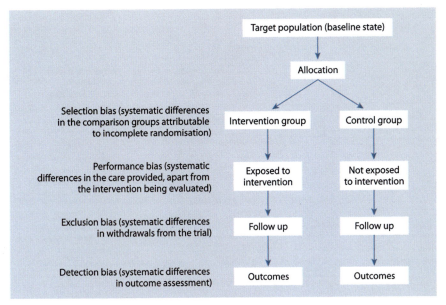

■ **Fig. 5.1** Possible sources of bias to look out for in randomized controlled clinical trials (RCTs). (Greenhalgh 1997)

■ Table 5.2 shows that bias factors of internal as well as of external validity can increase the tendency towards false-positive or false-negative results; they should therefore be individually assessed for each study.

Due to their basic design the various types of trials also hold the potential for different bias tendencies. As was mentioned earlier, the RCT design (with high internal validity, including blinding and ITT analysis) is chosen primarily to avoid false-positive results, but it does render the study more susceptible to false-negative results.

The following factors may provoke false-negative results in RCTs:

- Treatment errors, wrong dosage
- Adjuvant and compensatory treatment (of side effects etc.)
- Specific effects of 'placebo' treatment
- Dropouts and non-compliers
- Contamination (patients in placebo group receive effective interventions) and intention-to-treat analysis
- Informed consent (with the fear of not receiving optimal treatment)
- Obsequiousness bias, experimental subordination
- Poor differentiating power of the assessment method
- Central tendency bias; group assimilation
- Pitfalls during patient recruitment
- Conditioning effects
- Cognitive interactions
- Disturbance of the physician-patient relationship
- Simplified study design (mega-studies)
  (adapted from Kienle 2005)

5

❑ Table 5.2 Bias factors that may affect internal and external validity*			
Bias factors		**Internal validity**	**External validity / generalisability**
Selection bias	problem	verum and control group are not comparable in terms of age, severity of illness	study population is not representative; study population and 'target population' are not comparable; differences in age, severity of illness, for example
	possible solutions	randomisation, matched-pair analysis	comparison of epidemiological and study- relevant factors (also risk factors), also with patients who did not assent to the study
	false-negative/ -positive results possible due to:	$\ominus$: relevant subgroup differentiations are not known → levelling out of effect $\oplus$: e.g. more responders in the verum group	$\oplus/\ominus$: e.g. study group with higher illness severity grade (e.g. in university clinics) $\oplus$: no concomitant conditions that complicate treatment (exclusion criterion)
	key questions	Is randomisation adequate? Are relevant factors such as concomitant diseases documented?	Were epidemiological and study-relevant factors taken into account?
Performance bias	problem	groups are treated differently (beyond the test intervention)	study intervention does not reflect individual treatment variability under real practice conditions
	possible solutions	blinding (double or single), documentation of potential differences, change to open-label design (COLA)	authentic treatment variability and, if applicable, modification (pragmatic controlled trials)
	false-negative/ -positive results possible due to:	$\ominus$: additional (self-) medication in control group; non-compliance in verum group; $\oplus$: additional effective self-medication in verum group	$\oplus$: (too) high compliance (hospital treatment) and specialist physicians, dosage too high; $\ominus$: relevant context factors are lacking, e.g. physician-patient interaction based on trust, inexperienced physicians, dosage too low
	key questions:	Is blinding adequate and was it checked during the study? Is there documentation of concomitant intervention?	Are the interventions executed 'true to reality' by the same physicians as under practice conditions?
Attrition bias	problem	dropout rates in groups differ, which makes evaluation unreliable	dropout rates between study and target population differ, e.g. due to different motivation, compliance, feasibility
▼	possible solutions	intention-to-treat analysis (ITT); NB: drop-out rate >10% involves higher bias risk	compliance control and evaluation

☐ **Table 5.2** (continued)

Bias factors		Internal validity	External validity / generalisability
	false-negative/ -positive results possible due to:	⊖: ITT analyses; ⊕: per-protocol analysis (PP) with higher dropout rate in verum group	⊖: dropouts due to unexpected events (and ITT analysis); ⊕: dropouts due to ineffective treatment (and PP analysis)
	key questions	Was the dropout rate documented? Were adequate analyses (ITT and PP) carried out?	Were dropout causes documented? Do the causes for dropping out affect evaluation of effectiveness, compliance or safety of treatment?
Detection bias	problem	differences in perception/ assessment of outcome parameters between groups or in the course of the study (before-after comparison)	Chosen end points and/or observation period do not reflect the 'actual' relevant disease process.
	possible solutions	blinding of evaluators, objectifiable parameters; two independent evaluators	selection of clinically and practice-relevant end points, sufficiently long follow-up
	false-negative/ -positive results possible due to:	⊖/⊕: lack of or insufficient blinding with corresponding expectations on the part of the evaluator	⊖: end points do not reflect actual treatment success; inadequate observation period; ⊕: result significant but clinically irrelevant
	key questions	blinded evaluator? independent evaluators?	Were end points, observation period and established differences clinically and practically relevant?

* ⊖/⊕ factors shown are examples that do not necessarily bias the result in the direction indicated: in the interaction between physician and patient 'nocebo effects' are also possible.

In observational studies, controlled studies with COLA (Change to Open Label) design (de-blinding possible if wished by patient or physician and included in the evaluation, cf. Hogel et al. 1994) or pragmatic controlled trials (treatment variabilities and modification are possible, documented and included in the evaluation, cf. Roland and Torgerson 1998, Resch 1998, Godwin et al. 2003), one tries to achieve high external validity, although in most cases this goes with a tendency to false-positive results due to 'selective perception' and, for studies without control, due to mistaken causality (e.g. of regression-towards-the-mean phenomena).

One can also conclude from this that positive results in RCTs and probably also negative results in observational studies are on the whole more reliable than the other way around (i.e. negative RCT results and positive observational studies). RCTs have the advantage of being able to trace back the outcome with high probability to the test intervention, but, due to their experimental design, they suppress important factors that are crucial for effectiveness. Non-RCTs, in contrast, are able to incorporate relevant contextual factors such as patient preferences and individual treatment modifications and are consequently more true to actual practice.

Their disadvantage is that they cannot necessarily and with certainty trace the outcome back to the investigational intervention.

The single-case analysis has the potential to show up a specific causality very clearly (not to be confused with $n=1$ studies which use randomisation).

With the appropriate correspondence patterns (see below) this causality becomes apparent, but documentation has to be meticulous to avoid over-interpretation and selective perception.

The following aspects are relevant: (adapted from Kienle et al. 2004):

- Was the diagnosis confirmed by state-of-the-art means?
- Was the relevant baseline information documented (the study's reference points and end points; age, gender, pre-/post-menopausal, general state of health, risk factors and other relevant medical information)?
- Was the intervention sufficiently and comprehensibly documented (e.g. accurate product names, dosage, form and frequency of application, treatment modification if applicable)?
- Is there information regarding unexpected adverse events (UAE) (tolerability, side effects)?
- Was the main end point (and any subsidiary end points) well chosen (e.g. does it truly reflect the treatment expectation)?
- Was the method for determining the main end point (and any subsidiary goals) well chosen?
- Was the length of time for the determination of the main end point (and any subsidiary end points) well chosen?
- Was the outcome confirmed by a neutral second person?
- Were dropouts registered (with study-relevant reasons if applicable)?
- Is the process, especially the temporal relationship between intervention and outcome, clearly and comprehensibly described?
- Is there information regarding confounding factors: adjuvant and prior treatment (what? when? for how long? how much? by whom? to what effect?), co-morbidities or other changes in state of health during treatment, change of lifestyle (incl. change of residence or partner, holiday, changes in diet or exercise)?
- Can the outcome be attributed to the intervention according to CBM (cognition-based medicine) criteria? CBM criteria (adapted from Kiene 2001) are:
  - before/after temporal relationship (weakest criterion because other influences can never be entirely excluded)
  - correspondence of temporal patterns
  - correspondence of spatial patterns
  - morphological correspondence
  - dose-effect correspondence
  - process correspondence
  - dialogue correspondence
  - functional causal *gestalt*
  - functional therapeutic process
  What level of certainty applies to the grading (likely, possible, unlikely)?
- How many patients in comparable situations did not receive the intervention (and why?) or had a different outcome?

Ideally, the single-case analysis can assign a relatively specific correspondence of intervention and effect, just like the RCT albeit in a different way. However, it does not provide information on the frequency with which the effect will occur in a possible target population. In other words, it can demonstrate potential effectiveness but not 'real-world effectiveness'.

Unlike systematic reviews (SR) and meta-analyses (MA), HTAs focus mainly on assessing 'real-world effectiveness', which is the effectiveness in the every-day practice situation, while the specificity of the effect, which is the chief concern of SR and MA, is of secondary importance. In order to assess and evaluate real-world effectiveness the present HTA examined the studies also for criteria of external validity (see ◘ Tables 5.3–5.7, excerpts from data extraction forms; for complete form see appendix):

Documentation, internal and external validity were evaluated in three stages (◘ Table 5.8); the relationship between validity criteria, bias, validity evaluation and result interpretation was based on Alderson et al. (2004).

The two categories 'one or more criteria partly met' and 'one or more criteria not met' seem identical at first glance. What is meant is probably that, as soon as one criterion is not met, a high risk of bias is assumed – without validation of the criteria. The specification 'all of the criteria met' can also be realistically and meaningfully applied only to evaluation systems that include few criteria, all of which should be equally relevant, such as the Jadad Score for internal validity. For comprehensive assessment tools such as the questionnaires of the present HTA, classification according to SIGN 50 is more practicable (◘ Table 5.9):

The ratings 'low', 'moderate' or 'high risk of bias' or overall results of ++, + or – correspond to the grades good, moderate and poor validity.

◘ Table 5.3 Population

Was diagnosis established in line with the medical speciality?	☐ yes	☐ no	☐ n/a
Adjuvant medication (during the trial)?	comments:		
Is the population relevant to the question of this particular study?	☐ yes ☐ no comments:	☐ partly ☐ not clear	
Are duration and severity as well as co-morbidity and prognostic factors mentioned?			

◘ Table 5.4 Study design/methods

Is the study design adequate for the speciality?	☐ yes ☐ not clear comments:	☐ partly	☐ no

◘ Table 5.5 Intervention

Was the intervention correctly implemented (in line with the medical speciality)?	☐ yes ☐ no comments:	☐ partly ☐ ?

5

◘ Table 5.6 End points and outcomes

end point relevant to investigational condition?	☐ yes ☐ to an extent ☐ no ☐ ?
Is there adequate documentation of unexpected adverse events (UAE)/side effects?	☐ yes ☐ to an extent ☐ no ☐ not documented
results for UAE/side effects	++ statistically significant increase in UAEs with test intervention + tendency to increase with test intervention (trend) +/- no difference - trend for control treatment -- statistical significance for control treatment ∅ no UAEs observed n.d.: not documented
Comments on determination of end point (measuring method: validity and significance of end point)	

◘ Table 5.7 Questions specific to homeopathy

treatment based on similarity rule	☐ yes ☐ to an extent (e.g. complex remedies) ☐ no ☐ not documented
therapeutic concept	☐ individual homeopathy ☐ clinical homeopathy ☐ complex homeopathy ☐ isopathy ☐ not documented
weight of symptoms (hierarchisation/repertorisation) documented	☐ yes ☐ no
confounding factors taken into account	☐ yes ☐ no
Was evaluation of homeopathic responses and results based on homeopathic criteria?	☐ yes ☐ no
comments: (aspects of specialisation)	

◘ Table 5.8 Relationship between risk of bias, interpretation of results and validity criteria (Alderson et al. 2004)

Risk of bias	Interpretation	Relationship to individual criteria
A – low risk of bias	plausible bias unlikely to seriously alter the results	all of the criteria met
B – moderate risk of bias	plausible bias that raises some doubt about the results	one or more criteria partly met
C – high risk of bias	plausible bias that seriously weakens confidence in the results	one or more criteria not met

☑ **Table 5.9** Relationship between validity criteria, risk of bias of the study outcome and overall evaluation according to SIGN 50 (2004)	
++	**All or most** of the criteria have been fulfilled. Where they have not been fulfilled the conclusions of the study or review are thought <u>very unlikely</u> to alter.
+	**Some** of the criteria have been fulfilled. Those criteria that have not been fulfilled or not adequately described are thought <u>unlikely</u> to alter the conclusions.
-	**Few or no** criteria fulfilled. The conclusions of the study are thought <u>likely or very likely</u> to alter.

In our HTA, real-world effectiveness was then evaluated in a three-stage process as a synthesis of outcome significance, quality and frequency of observations:

1. Effectiveness is likely if there are significant and broader positive trend results in good quality trials (i.e. low or moderate risk of confounding through bias factors that are internally and externally valid).
2. Effectiveness is questionable, e.g., if there are only single case reports and no collective studies of acceptable quality.
3. Effectiveness is unlikely if there are only positive single case reports and negative collective studies of acceptable quality.

5.3 Problems with the Formal Evaluation of Clinical Trials in Meta-analyses

The danger of biased evaluation due to one-sided focus on purely formal criteria without thematic differentiation has been confirmed in the PEK project. The research team led by Matthias Egger at the Institute for Social and Preventive Medicine at the University of Bern was commissioned by the PEK steering committee to examine the quality of clinical trials that compare homeopathy, traditional Chinese medicine (TCM) and phytotherapy with conventional medicine. A total of 110 clinical homeopathic studies were systematically identified and compared (in terms of indication and end points) with corresponding studies of conventional medicine. There were more high-quality studies for homeopathy (21 studies) than for conventional medicine (eight studies)! Of these, the studies with a larger sample size or lower standard deviation (exact criteria were unfortunately not mentioned) were used to determine a combined effect value for the medical approach in question. The six conventional medicine studies had an odds ratio (OR) of 0.58 (95% CI 0.39–0.85), which suggests effectiveness as the confidence interval (CI) was below 1, while the eight homeopathy studies had an odds ratio of 0.88 (95% CI 0.65–1.19). In addition, all studies were entered into a funnel plot which displayed asymmetry for homeopathy as well as for conventional medicine. This was interpreted for both as being due to bias (publication bias and similar) as the heterogeneity of the studies was considered to be responsible for 'only' 65% (homeopathy) or 77% (conventional medicine) of the variability (I^2 values based on Higgins and Thompson 2002). From the authors' point of view, the result was compatible with the thesis that the clinical effects of homeopathy are placebo effects (Shang et al. 2005a).

The Lancet editorial entitled 'The end of homeopathy' went even further: 'Surely the time has passed for selective analyses, biased reports, or further investment in research to perpetuate the homeopathy versus allopathy debate. Now doctors need to be bold and honest with their patients about homeopathy's lack of benefit, and with themselves about the failings of modern medicine to address patients' needs for personalized care' (Editorial Lancet 2005).

Leaving aside the lack of fair play, the conclusion as it stands is not correct because it applies to placebo-controlled trials as well – although they rarely show significance for placebo – that 'absence of evidence' is not the same as 'evidence of absence' (Altman and Bland 1995).

The study attracted criticism from various other sides:

- The authors did not adhere to the QUORUM guidelines regarding the conducting of meta-analyses which stipulate descriptive data as well as data for the evaluation of effect values and confidence intervals for the studies that are being investigated. 'The lack of detail is unacceptable in a paper drawing a strong clinical conclusion' (Linde and Jonas 2005).
- The extent to which the selected studies are representative of homeopathic practice (i.e. externally valid) has not been explained (Walach et al. 2005a).
- Combining outcome data makes sense only if the different trials are measuring the same effect. If homeopathy, for instance, helps with some conditions and not with others (cf. Jonas et al. 2003) a funnel plot cannot be evaluated and a combined effect value is meaningless (Linde and Jonas 2005).
- The assumption that the effect size is the same for all placebo-control groups is probably not tenable either; CAM therapies appear to have a high placebo responder rate in general, so that the placebo effect in homeopathic studies lies partly above the treatment effect of conventional interventions (a phenomenon known as the Walach efficacy paradox, 2001, quoted from Walach et al. 2005a). In conventional medicine trials the so-called placebo effect also varies strongly (Walach et al. 2005b).
- Because the sample size depends on disease, intervention and chosen outcome, an analysis that is restricted to large trials harbours the risk of false-negative results. It is therefore not possible to differentiate between the dependencies mentioned and a genuine bias (Linde and Jonas 2005).
- As the main conclusion relies on six or eight trials ('probably unmatched'), the result could easily be due to chance, which would also explain the high confidence interval (Linde and Jonas 2005).

Skandhan et al. (2005) published a remarkable comment which reflects the outcry the study and the editorial provoked in India. Homeopathy is widespread there and highly valued by the population as well as by allopathic physicians and the institutions / authorities in charge. It is supported by the World Health Organisation. The state secretary for Ayurveda, homeopathy and yoga, Uma Pillai, commented: 'How could a single study dismiss an entire system?'

We share most of the concerns presented here and support in particular the criticism that external validity and model validity are not given sufficient consideration.

Table 5.10 shows that – in accordance with the claim of Linde and Jonas (2005) – the trials used to determine the combined effect value show only one incidence of insufficient matching:

Ten conditions were investigated, of which only two were covered by both conventional and homeopathic studies: influenza and diarrhoea. Both showed significant effects for both the homeopathic and the conventional medical intervention. The homeopathic study registered fewer side effects, which confirms a comment made by Raoult (2005), an allopath, who, in line with the ancient maxim of *primum non nocere* (first, do no harm) sees in homeopathy a serious alternative to conventional medicine.

Table 5.10 Disorders and relevant high-quality studies (based on Shang et al. 2005a,b)

Indication	Conventional medicine		Homeopathy	
	Study	Result	Study	Result
post-abortal bacterial vaginosis	Crowley et al. 2001; antibiotic prophylaxis	n.s.		
stroke	Horn et al. 2001; nimodipine treatment	n.s.		
allergic conjunctivitis	Möller et al. 1994; treatment with nedocromil (children); significant in 2 of 3 parameters; high placebo effect	sign.		
influenza	De Flora et al. 1997: prophylactic treatment with N-acetyl-cysteine; significant attenuation of symptoms; pathogen equally detectable in both groups	sign.		
	Nicholson 2000: treatment with oseltamivir	sign.	Papp et al. 1998: treatment with Oscillococcinum®	sign.
			Rottey et al. 1995: treatment with micro-organisms	sign.
acute diarrhoea (children)	Kaplan et al. 1999: treatment with loperamide; high rate of side effects	sign.	Jacobs et al. 2000: treated with homeopathic medicines; children in Nepal; few side effects	sign.
headache			Walach et al. 1997: classical homeopathy	n.s.
chron. sinusitis			Weiser and Clasen 1994: complex – Euphorbium comp.	sign.
warts			Labrecque et al. 1992: homeopathic treatment; endpoint: total elimination of warts	n.s.
muscle soreness			Vickers et al. 1998: prophylactic Arnica D30 (after long-distance running)	n.s. (trend for placebo)
support during fasting			Schmidt and Ostermayr 2002: supporting weight reduction in fasting patients with Thyroidinum C30	n.s. (trend for placebo; significance without adjustment)

n.s. – not significant; sign. – significant
A more detailed account of homeopathic effectiveness for the health problems mentioned can be found in Lüdtke (2006).

Homeopaths will find the non-significant results of the muscle soreness and fasting studies, which even show a clear trend for placebo, hardly surprising. Both studies are experimental in character and have very little external validity for the homeopathic practice. The muscle soreness that occurred after prophylactic application of Arnica (after long-distance-running, before the muscle soreness was expected to set in) can certainly be interpreted as drug proving, and the absence of weight loss with Thyroidinum during fasting as a 'therapeutic' effect in line with the similarity principle. If we remove both studies from the evaluation because of their low external validity we end up with a much higher effectiveness for homeopathy that is almost comparable to that of conventional medicine.

Yet, no comparison with conventional medicine is necessary to prove the effectiveness of homeopathy. It merely serves to illustrate the absurdity of the procedure, i.e. the non-comparability (of treatments for stroke and warts).

(Among the 110 conventional medical studies there are also some that are based on homeopathic thinking such as 'The safety and efficacy of subcutaneous birch pollen immunotherapy', 'Conservative treatment of chronic sinusitis – success of oral bacterial lysate therapy' or 'Oral immunotherapy in birch pollen hay fever').

The comparability of the trials is essential for a meaningful and fair comparison. In order to determine a combined-effect value one therefore uses the fixed-effect model if a uniform effect size can be expected, with deviations being caused only by measuring inaccuracies; the random-effect model is used if one expects population variance on top of the measuring deviation whilst assuming normal distribution. If these conditions are met, a combined-effect value can be determined and a symmetrical funnel plot can be expected or any asymmetry can be attributed to publication or other bias. If that is not the case, the most common cause for an asymmetrical funnel plot lies in the heterogeneity of the trials. The direction of the asymmetry is also predetermined: the smaller the effect, the larger the population must be in order to allow for effect differentiation (cf. also Penston 2005 and Linde and Jonas 2005).

In his 1997 meta-analysis, Linde explained the combination of individual study effect sizes into a combined-effect value with his null hypothesis: homeopathic remedies = placebo with a uniform effect size being expected (Linde and Jonas 2005). Linde's approach provoked much criticism at the time. As mentioned earlier, Walach (2001) also referred to possible 'efficacy paradoxes' for CAM therapies, so that one cannot even assume a uniform effect size for placebo. The effect size, or rather its determination, is dependent not only on the intervention, but also on an organism's responsiveness, the disease and its duration, the selected population, other contextual factors and on the measuring method applied. The negative result of an asthma trial (White et al. 2003), for example, was interpreted as a 'ceiling' effect when analysed in more detail (Fisher et al. 2005), which means that either the population was too 'sick', the test intervention was confounded by other interventions or factors, or the measuring method was calibrated down to adequately reflect the changes that 'normally' occur (external validity). It is, by the way, not to be expected that a conventional medical diagnosis will 'unify' the effect size of a homeopathic treatment, as that depends to a much higher degree on factors such as individual responsiveness than on the supposed laws of a disease process derived from collective figures.

Because of the extreme heterogeneity ($I^2 \geq 60\%$) of the studies by Shang et al. (2005a), funnel plotting as well as combined effect values are difficult. 'It's important to remember that whatever statistical model you choose, you have to be confident that clinical and methodological diversity is not so great that we should not be combining studies at all.' (http://www.cochrane-net.org/openlearning/HTML/mod13-4.htm – quoted from Cochrane 'Textbook').

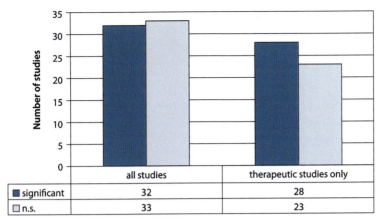

	all studies	therapeutic studies only
■ significant	32	28
□ n.s.	33	23

Fig. 5.2 Comparison of significant and non-significant results of all studies on homeopathy with those of purely therapeutic studies. The values for the study results that were also used by Shang et al. (2005a) are taken from Linde et al (1997) (as Shang and al. did not provide figures). Not all studies by Shang et al. could therefore be included in the diagram

The reference list of 220 studies in Shang et al. (2005a) includes more than 60 different conditions from allergic asthma, anal fissures and anxiety through gastritis, brain trauma, postoperative complications and prevention (mostly of infections) to varices and warts. Only 14 conditions appear more than once. Furthermore, there are differences concerning the populations tested (children/adults), duration and kinds of illness (acute, chronic) etc. If one compares the studies that are actually comparable – same/comparable population, same intervention and same end points and testing as was the case with irritable colon, diarrhoea and pollinosis (data based on Linde et al. 1997) the results contradict the conclusions of Shang et al. (2005a). The higher the number of cases (or: the smaller the confidence interval), the more favourable the result for homeopathy. There is even a 'symmetric' funnel plot for the four pollinosis studies.

This evidence proves that differentiation in terms of content is essential. As mentioned earlier in this chapter, ignoring EV and MV can also affect the result. It is not just a question of whether classical homeopathy was used or not, but also of whether modifications of homeopathic remedies were permitted, the homeopaths were experienced enough, the follow-up period was long enough, or Hering's Law or initial aggravation could be included in the evaluation of pathological processes. Without more detailed knowledge of the 110 studies it is not possible to decide whether the analysis would yield a different overall conclusion if these external validity criteria were taken into account. Removing the prevention studies – which are unusual in homeopathy – from the comparison certainly changes the ratio of significant and non-significant studies (see ◻ Fig. 5.2), although a vote count is not adequate for a synthesis of results (see Chaps. 9.4.4 and 13).

In summary, we can say that there is a considerable risk of bias if formal criteria are overrated and there is no differentiation of content or consideration of external validity and model validity criteria, as is frequently the case with meta-analyses. Due to retrospective selection and lack of confounder control, meta-analyses are also not protected against overt or hidden bias. 'If one evaluated an RCT with these means, it would fail the Cochrane test' (Wegscheider 2005; cf. also Chap. 13, p 221).

While the above argument does not allow us to draw the reverse conclusion that homeopathy is effective, it does support the claim that the Shang et al. study (2005a) does not prove the ineffectiveness of homeopathy. In view of the obvious error potential of that study, one can only concur with Uma Pillai: 'How could a single study dismiss an entire system?' (Skandhan et al. 2005).

5.4   References

Agency for Health Care Policy and Research (AHCPR). Acute pain management: operative and medical procedures and trauma. Clinical practice guideline No.1. AHCPR Publication 1992 No. 92-0023, Appendix B. available at: http://www.ncbi.nlm.nih.gov/books/bv.fcgi?rid=hstat6.table.9286

Alderson P, Green S, Higgins J (2004)Cochrane Reviewers' Handbook. Handbook 4.2.1. [updated December 2003]. John Wiley & Sons Ltd, Chichester

Altman DG, Bland JM (1995) Absence of evidence is not evidence of absence. BMJ 311:485

Bornhöft G, Maxion-Bergemann S, Wolf U, Kienle G, Michalsen A, Vollmar H, Gilbertson S, Matthiessen P (2006) Checklist for the qualitative evaluation of clinical studies with particular focus on external validity and model validity. BMC Med Res Methodol 6:56

Bundesamt für Sozialversicherung der Schweiz (ed) (1996)Handbuch zur Standardisierung der medizinischen und wirtschaftlichen Bewertung medizinischer Leistungen, 3rd edn. Bern

Cochrane Collaboration (2002) The Cochrane Collaboration open learning material. 13: Diversity and heterogeneity. Available at: http://www.cochrane-net.org/openlearning/HTML/mod13-4.htm

Crowley T, Low N, Turner A, Harvey I, Bidgood K, Horner P (2001) Antibiotic prophylaxis to prevent post-abortal upper genital tract infection in women with bacterial vaginosis: randomized controlled trial. BJOG Int J Obstet Gynaecol 108:396–402

De Flora S, Grassi C, Carati L (1997) Attenuation of influenza-like symptomatology and improvement of cell-mediated immunity with long-term N-acetylcysteine treatment. Eur Respir J 10:1535–1541

Dickersin K (2003) The mammography debate: a crisis for evidence-based medicine? In: 4. Symposion Evidenzbasierte Medizin. 14–15 March, 2003,Freiburg i.Br.

Editorial (2005) The end of homeopathy. Lancet 366:690; DOI:10.1016/S0140-6736(05)67149-8

Ernst E (2004) Author's reply. Wien Klin Wochenschr 116:408

Fisher P, Berman B, Davidson J, Reilly D, Thompson T (2005) Are the clinical effects of homeopathy placebo effects? Lancet 366:2082–2083; DOI:10.1016/S0140-6736(05)67879-8

Gill P, Dowell AC, Neal RD, Smith N, Heywood P, Wilson AE (1996) Evidence-based general practice: a retrospective study of interventions in one training practice. BMJ 312:819–821

Godwin M, Ruhland L, Casson I, MacDonald S, Delva D, Birtwhistle R, Lam M, Seguin R (2003) Pragmatic controlled clinical trials in primary care: the struggle between external and internal validity. BMC Med Res Methodol 3:28. DOI:10.1186/1471-2288-3-28

Greenhalgh T (1997) Assessing the methodological quality of published papers. BMJ 315:305–308

Habour R, Miller J (2001) A new system for grading recommendations in evidence based guidelines. BMJ 323:334–336

Heusser P (2001) Kriterien zur Beurteilung des Nutzens von komplementärmedizinischen Methoden. Forschende Komplementärmedizin und Klassische Naturheilkunde 8:14–23

Higgins JPT, Thompson SG (2002) Quantifying heterogeneity in a meta-analysis. Stat Med 21:1539–1558

Hogel J, Walach H, Gaus W (1994) Change-to-Open-Label Design. Proposal and discussion of a new design for clinical parallel-group double-masked trials. Arzneimittelforschung 44:97–99

Horn J, de Haan RJ, Vermeulen M, Limburg M (2001) Very early nimodipine use in stroke (VENUS): a randomized, double-blind, placebo-controlled trial. Stroke 32:461–465

Jacobs J, Jimenez LM, Malthouse S, Chapman E, Crothers D, Masuk M, Jonas WB (2000) Homeopathic treatment of acute childhood diarrhea: results from a clinical trial in Nepal. J Altern Complement Med 6:131–139

Jonas WB, Kaptchuk TJ, Linde K (2003) A critical overview of homeopathy. Ann Intern Med 138:393–399

Kaplan MA, Prior MJ, McKonly KI, DuPont HL, Temple AR, Nelson EB (1999) A multicenter randomized controlled trial of a liquid loperamide product versus placebo in the treatment of acute diarrhea in children. Clin Pediatr 38:579–591

Khan KS, ter Riet G, Popay J, Nixon J, Kleijnen J (2001) STAGE II – Conducting the review. PHASE 5 – Study quality assessment. In: Khan KS, ter Riet G, Glanville J, Sowden AJ, Kleijnen J (eds) Undertaking systematic reviews of research on effectiveness. CRD Report Number 4 (2nd edn), York

Kiene H (2001) Komplementäre Methodenlehre der klinischen Forschung. Cognition-based Medicine. Springer, Berlin Heidelberg New York

Kienle G (1974) Arzneimittelsicherheit und Gesellschaft. Eine kritische Untersuchung. Schattauer, Stuttgart New York

Kienle GS (2005) Gibt es Gründe für Pluralistische Evaluationsmodelle? Limitationen der Randomisierten Klinischen Studie. Z Arztl Fortbild Qualität Gesundheitswesen 99:289–294

Kienle GS, Hamre HJ, Portalupi E, Kiene H (2004) Improving the quality of therapeutic reports of single cases and case series in oncology – criteria and checklist. Altern Therapies Health Med 10:68–72

Kienle GS, Kiene H, Albonico HU (2006a) Anthroposophische Medizin in der klinischen Forschung. Schattauer, Stuttgart New York

Kienle GS, Kiene H, Albonico HU (2006b)Anthroposophic medicine. Effectiveness, utility, costs, safety. Schattauer, Stuttgart New York

Labrecque M, Audet D, Latulippe LG, Drouin J (1992) Homeopathic treatment of plantar warts. Can Med Assoc J 146:1749–1753

Linde K, Clausius N, Ramirez G, Melchart D, Eitel F, Hedges LV, Jonas WB (1997) Are the clinical effects of homeopathy placebo effects? A meta-analysis of placebo-controlled trials. Lancet 350:834–843

Linde K, Jonas W (2005) Are the clinical effects of homeopathy placebo effects? Lancet 366:2081–2082; DOI:10.1016/S0140-6736(05)67878-6

Lüdtke R (ed) (2006) Homöopathie – Zum Stand der klinischen Forschung. Eine Stellungnahme der Karl und Veronica Carstens-Stiftung. KVC, Essen. available at: www.carstens-stiftung.de/wissen/hom/pdf/Stand_der_Forschung_Homeopathie_07MAR06.pdf

Matthiessen PF (2003) Der diagnostisch-therapeutische Prozess als Problem der Einzelfallforschung. In: Ostermann T, Matthiessen PF (eds) Einzelfallforschung in der Medizin. Bedeutung, Möglichkeiten, Grenzen. VAS, Frankfurt

Matthiessen PF (2005) Die Therapieentscheidung des Arztes. Z Arztl Fortbild Qualität Gesundheitswesen 99:269–273

Moher D, Cook DJ, Jadad AR, Tugwell P, Moher M, Jonas A, Pham B, Klassen TP (1999) Assessing the quality of reports of randomized trials: implications for the conduct of meta-analyses. Health Technol Assess 3:i–iv, 1–98

Moller C, Berg IM, Berg T, Kjellman M, Stromberg L (1994) Nedocromil sodium 2% eye drops for twice-daily treatment of seasonal allergic conjunctivitis: a Swedish multicentre placebo-controlled study in children allergic to birch pollen. Clin Exp Allergy 24:884–887

Nicholson KG, Aoki FY, Osterhaus AD, Trottier S, Carewicz O, Mercier CH, Rode A, Kinnersley N, Ward P (2000) Efficacy and safety of oseltamivir in treatment of acute influenza: a randomized controlled trial. Neuraminidase Inhibitor Flu Treatment Investigator Group. Lancet 355:1845–1850

Niroomand F (2004) Evidenzbasierte Medizin: das Individuum bleibt auf der Strecke. Dtsch Ärztebl 101:1870–1874

Ollenschläger G, Helou A, Lorenz W (2000) Kritische Bewertung von Leitlinien. In: Kunz R, Ollenschläger G, Raspe HH (eds). Lehrbuch evidenzbasierte Medizin in Klinik und Praxis. Schriftenreihe Hans Neuffer Stiftung. Deutscher ÄrzteVerlag, Köln, pp 156–176

Papp R, Schuback G, Beck E, Burkard G, Bengel J, Lehrl S, Belon P (1998) Oscillococcinum® in patients with influenza-like syndromes: a placebo-controlled double-blind evaluation. Br Homeopathic J 87:69–76

Penston J (2005) Large-scale randomized trials – a misguided approach to clinical research. Med Hypotheses 64:651–657

Raoult D (2005) Are the clinical effects of homeopathy placebo effects? Authors' reply. Lancet 366:2085–2086; DOI:10.1016/S0140-6736(05)67883-X

Resch K (1998) Pragmatic randomized controlled trials for complex therapies. Forschende Komplementärmedizin. 5 [Suppl S1]:S136–139

Roland M, Torgerson DJ (1998) Understanding controlled trials: What are pragmatic trials? BMJ 316:285

Rottey E, Verleye G, Liagre R (1995) Het effect van een homeopathische bereiding van micro-organismen bij de preventie van griepsymptomen: een gerandomiseered dubbel-blind onderzoek in de huisartspraktijk. Tijdschr Integrale Geneeskunde 11:54–58

Sackett D, Richardson W, Haynes R (1997) Evidence-based medicine. How to practice and teach EBM. Churchill Livingstone, New York Edinburgh London

Sackett DL (1979) Bias in analytic research. J Chronic Dis 32:51–63

Schmidt JM, Ostermayr B (2002) Does a homeopathic ultramolecular dilution of Thyroidinum 30cH affect the rate of body weight reduction in fasting patients? A randomized placebo-controlled double-blind clinical trial. Homeopathy 91:197–206

Shang A, Huwiler-Muntener K, Nartey L, Jüni P, Dörig S, Sterne JAC, Pewsner D, Egger M (2005a) Are the clinical effects of homeopathy placebo effects? Comparative study of placebo-controlled trials of homeopathy and allopathy. Lancet 366:726–732; DOI:10.1016/S0140-6736(05)67177-2

Shang a, Jüni P, Sterne JAC, Huwiler-Müntener K, Egger M (2005b) Are the clinical effects of homeopathy placebo effects? Authors' reply. Lancet 366:2083–2085; DOI:10.1016/S0140-6736(05)67881-6

SIGN 50 (Scottish Intercollegiate Guidelines Network). A guideline developer's handbook. Notes on the use of Methodology Checklist 2: Randomized Controlled Trials. available at: http://www.sign.ac.uk/guidelines/fulltext/50/notes2.html

Skandhan KP, Smith A, Avni A (2005) Are the clinical effects of homeopathy placebo effects? Authors' reply. Lancet 366:2085; DOI:10.1016/S0140-6736(05)67882-8

Vickers AJ, Fisher P, Smith C, Wyllie SE, Rees R (1998) Homeopathic Arnica 30x is ineffective for muscle soreness after long-distance running: a randomized, double-blind, placebo-controlled trial. Clin J Pain 14:227–231

Walach H, Haeusler W, Lowes T, Mussbach D, Schamell U, Springer W, Stritzl G, Gaus W, Haag G (1997) Classical homeopathic treatment of chronic headaches. Cephalalgia 17:119–126; discussion: p 101

Walach H, Jonas W, Lewith G (2005a) Are the clinical effects of homeopathy placebo effects? Lancet 366:2081; DOI:10.1016/S0140-6736(05)67877-4)

Walach H, Sadaghiani C, Dehm C, Bierman DJ (2005b) The therapeutic effect of clinical trials: understanding placebo response rates in clinical trials – a secondary analysis. BMC Med Res Methodol 5:26

Walach H (2001) Das Wirksamkeitsparadox in der Komplementärmedizin. Forschende Komplementärmedizin und Klassische Naturheilkunde 8:193–195

Wegscheider K (2005) Was sind faire Vergleiche zwischen Therapien? Zeitschrift für ärztliche Fortbildung und Qualität im Gesundheitswesen 99:275–278

Wein C (2002)Qualitätsaspekte klinischer Studien zur Homöopathie. KVC, Essen

Weiser M, Clasen B (1994) Randomisierte plazebokontrollierte Doppelblindstudie zur Untersuchung der klinischen Wirksamkeit der homöopathischen Euphorbium compositum-Nasentropfen S bei chronischer Sinusitis. Forschende Komplementärmedizin 1:251–259

White A, Slade P, Hunt C, Hart A, Ernst E (2003) Individualized homeopathy as an adjunct in the treatment of childhood asthma: a randomized placebo controlled trial. Thorax 58:317–321

World Medical Association (2001) Declaration of Helsinki. Ethical principles for medical research involving human subjects. Bull World Health Organization, 79:373–374. available at: http://whqlibdoc.who.int/bulletin/2001/issue4/79(4)declaration.pdf

HTA Homeopathy: Methods and Material

Stefanie Maxion-Bergemann, Gudrun Bornhöft, Ursula Wolf

6.1   Project Implementation

The compilation of this HTA followed predefined steps to ensure the quality of process and results. The procedure was based on the commission documents provided and the generally accepted international guidelines for the compilation of HTA reports, as well as on the special requirements set by the 'Complementary Medicine Evaluation Programme' (PEK) in Switzerland (ECHTA 2001, BSV 2001, DIMDI 2004, INHTA 2001, Heusser 2001).

The project phases (for all research questions) were set out in an HTA protocol which was essentially adhered to. Any deviations and amendments are described in the text of the HTA report.

For the compilation of this HTA report the authors worked closely together with experts on methodology, specialist associations and expert advisers.

The latter were consulted on the following aspects:
- Search for relevant publications
- Specialized aspects of data extraction and evaluation of external validity for the published reviews and clinical trials on 'effectiveness'
- Selection of an indication ('domain') that could be representative for the investigation of 'effectiveness'
- Partly also data extraction and evaluation by experts in the relevant field
- Composition of specialized texts and chapter components
- Review of chapter components

The project proceeded in the following stages:
Scoping
- Defining the research question and establishing the methods for collecting the relevant data
- Searching various databases to identify the material available
- Contacting the specialist association and experts to agree on the above-mentioned aspects of collaboration

Focusing
- Preparing a questionnaire for data extraction and evaluation
- Review process with specialist associations and experts
- Establishing inclusion and exclusion criteria for the articles/titles found
- Deciding on suitable indications ('domains') in agreement with the specialist associations

To review all the data published in a specialist CAM field would exceed the margins of an HTA report. In collaboration with the experts an indication was therefore selected that was considered representative for the evaluation of effectiveness.

The following criteria were established for the **selection of such a representative indication:**
- The indication must be epidemiologically relevant, especially in Switzerland.
- Interventions must be comparable to those used in Switzerland.
- Studies must consider fundamental principles of the medical speciality.
- Interventions must be economically relevant.
- Sufficient publications must be available.

In addition, all systematic reviews and meta-analyses were checked for effectiveness and safety.

Procedure
- Systematic literature search
- Systematic review of publications
- Collection of further relevant information
- Synthesis of extracted data, evaluation and classification

Finalisation
- Compilation of HTA report and internal review process
- Submission of report with all its appendices to the PEK steering group in August 2004
- Review (by October 2004)
- Submission of final report with all its appendices to the PEK steering group in January 2005

6.2   Methods: Systematic Literature Search

Data collection:
The literature search served two general purposes which determined the choice of sources and the search strategy:
1. To provide an overview of accessible publications
2. To supply material on the basis of which the questions of the HTA could be answered

◘ Fig. 6.1 shows the sequence of steps for the literature search process.

6.2.1 Selection of data sources

The various data sources used to find the relevant material are briefly described in the next paragraph. Potential data sources to be searched were identified and selected primarily by screening the published reviews for the databases they had used (online libraries).

6.2.2 Data sources used

The following data sources were used:

Literature databases
In general, publically accessible (internet database providers) as well as non-public data collections were taken into account. ◘ Table 6.1 lists the databases including brief descriptions.

Internet resources
Apart from the literature databases there are various organisations that offer information via the Internet. Relevant information was obtained in this way mostly for the topics 'The Situation in Switzerland', 'General Information' and 'Methodology'. Access was via general Internet search engines. The sources used are included with the bibliographic references or appear with the

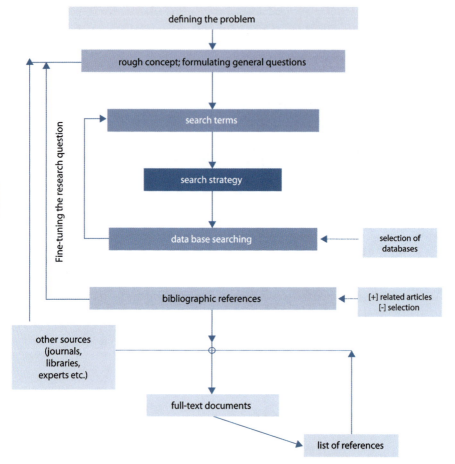

Fig. 6.1 Sequence of steps in the literature search process (adjusted from http://www.nlm.nih.gov/archive//2060905/nichsr/ehta/chapter4.html)

relevant quotations. The following sites were searched for HTA reports in the field of complementary medicine:

— Centre for Reviews and Dissemination, University of York, York, UK: http://www.york.ac.uk
— NHS R&D Health Technology Assessment Programme (NCCHTA) http://www.hta.nhsweb.nhs.uk
— International Network of Agencies for Health Technology Assessment (INHTA): a network of 42 HTA organisations (in North and Central America, Australia, New Zealand and Europe, founded in 1993)

Bibliographic references in articles
The bibliographic references in the articles that had been identified during stage one were then systematically screened for relevant publications.

For some specific questions manufacturers, experts etc. were contacted.

■ Table 6.1 Databases

Database	Time	Areas of focus	No. of journals	Provider
current contents/ clinical medicine	2002/wk 23– 2003/wk 22	cardiovascular and respiratory systems, clinical immunology and infectious disease, clinical psychology and psychiatry, dentistry/oral surgery and medicine, dermatology, endocrinology, metabolism and nutrition, environmental medicine and public health, gastroenterology and hepatology, general and internal medicine, health care sciences and services, hematology, neurology, oncology, ophthalmology, orthopaedics, rehabilitation and sports medicine, otolaryngology, paediatrics, pharmacology/ toxicology, radiology, nuclear medicine and imaging, reproductive medicine, research/laboratory medicine and medical technology, rheumatology, surgery, urology and nephrology	over 1120 journals and books	Institute for scientific information http://www.isinet.com/ journals/scope/ scope_cccm.html
dissertation abstracts	1990–May 2003	agriculture and food science, architecture, art, bioscience and biotechnology, business, chemistry, economics, education, history, geoscience, law and political science, mathematics, music, pharmaceuticals, psychology, social science, veterinary sciences, zoology	access to more than 90% of PhD dissertations (North America) Several thousand abstracts from other countries: more than 1.6 m medical dissertations	ProQuest Information and Learning; UMI Company, Ann Arbor, MI
EconlIt	1969–May 2003	international economics literature, from 1969	over 900; over 581,000 references	American Economic Association http://www.econlit.org
EMBASE	1980–2003/wk21	drug research, pharmacology, pharmaceutics, pharmacy, drug side effects and interactions, toxicology, human medicine (clinical and experimental), basic biological sciences, biotechnology, biomedical, medical devices, engineering and instrumentation, health policy and management, pharmaco-economics, public and occupational health, environmental health, pollution control, substance dependence and abuse, psychiatry, forensic science, alternative and complementary medicine, nursing	over 6500 titles from 70 countries; number of references: more than 16 titles	Elsevier

◘ Table 6.1 (continued)

Database	Time	Areas of focus	No. of journals	Provider
Evidence Based Medicine Reviews (EBMR): CDSR, ACP Journal Club, DARE, CCTR	until May 2003	resource for electronic information in the evidence-based medicine (EBM) movement that combines four of the most trusted EBM resources into a single, fully searchable database	over 360,000 references from to the following databases: CDSR (Cochrane Database of Systematic Reviews); ACP Journal Club (American College of Physicians); DARE (Database of Abstracts of Reviews of Effectiveness); CCTR (Cochrane Central Register of Clinical Trials)	American College of Physicians
AMED (Allied and Complementary Medicine)	1985–2003	alternative medicine	596; over 152,000 references	British Library
BIOSIS Previews	1969–2003/wk 23	biology, general; neuroscience; physiology; agronomy; biochemistry and biophysics; cell biology; genetics; zoology; multidisciplinary life and medical sciences; earth and environmental sciences; food science and technology; microbiology; anatomy; developmental biology; plant sciences; embryology; histology; molecular biology; neuroanatomy; pharmacology; science, general	more than 5000 international journals; 13,000,000 references	BIOSIS
CINAHL	1982–May 2003	professional literature of nursing, allied health, biomedicine and health care	1727; over 800,000 references	CINAHL Information Systems
Premedline + Medline	1966–May 2003	clinical medicine	ca. 4000; up to 11,800,000 references	U.S. National Library Medicine

6

Database	Date range	Content / subjects	References	Producer
PASCAL, BIOMED	1987–2003	multidisciplinary life and medical sciences/ subjects covered include applied biology; homeopathy; medicine; botany; science; pharmacology; toxicology; biotechnology; psychology etc.	more than 3100; 3,050,000 references	INIST-CNRS
PSYNDEXplus - Lit.& AV	1997–06/2003	records on psychology from researchers in Germany, Austria, and Switzerland	175,000 references	Institute for Psychology Information (ZPID) of the University of Trier/ Germany
SIGLE	1980–12/2002	European non-conventional ('grey') literature in the fields of pure and applied natural sciences and technology, economics, social sciences, and humanities	over 820,000 references	European Association for Grey Literature (EAGLE)
Social Sciences Full Text	1982–04/2003	addiction studies, anthropology, area studies, community health and medical care, corrections, criminal Justice, criminology, economics, environmental studies, ethics, family studies, gender studies, geography, gerontology, international relations, law, minority studies, planning and public administration, political science, psychiatry, psychology, public welfare, social work, sociology, urban studies	540; 750,000 references	H.W. Wilson Company

6.2.3   Systematic literature search: general search strategy and article selection

Search strategy (general)

1. A general extended search was conducted in online accessible databases (◻ Table 6.1) and all articles shown were saved to an internal database (Reference Manager Version 10). For the search strategy, possible search terms were decided upon and gradually extended and fine-tuned (◻ Fig. 6.1). The search strategy depended on the research question and also on the make-up of the databases to be searched. In general, a generic term was used for the specialisation and then coupled with additional search words for the respective questions. To cover different spellings of search terms as well as errors in the databases searched, truncations and wildcards such as 'hom?eopath$.af' were used.

2. In a second step, detailed electronic and manual searches (based on titles and abstracts) were carried out in the general database set up in step one.

3. Additional searches with special search terms were then conducted in the online databases to find articles that were relevant to individual questions.

4. The bibliographic references of all full-text articles were systematically screened (selection criteria as for 2 and 3).

The decision to obtain a full-text article for inclusion into the HTA depended on its potential relevance to one of the research questions (see Chap. 2.2).

For selecting articles that were to be ordered in full text the following **inclusion and exclusion criteria** were agreed:

- **Study design:** any study design that investigated the effectiveness/efficacy, use, safety or economy of an intervention
- **Population:** The populations and individual patients concerned had to be treated for therapeutic or prophylactic purposes.
- **Intervention:** any therapeutic or prophylactic intervention of the therapy approach under investigation
- **Comparison:** No restrictions applied regarding the treatment of the control group; i.e. placebo, conventional or complementary treatment were accepted.
- **Outcome:** Studies were included only if they investigated results that were relevant to patient care (i.e. parameters regarding therapeutic and prophylactic effectiveness, safety, use or economy).
- **Study status:** The study had to be published or an evaluable interim report had to be available.
- **Language:** The following languages were included for the PEK: English, German, Italian and French. (There was no language restriction for the database search, which means that relevant findings in other languages were also registered).

Review process for article selection:

The lists of articles were examined by two reviewers in the case of clinical studies and by one reviewer in the case of systematic reviews. Based on title and abstract (if available) the respective full-text articles were ordered.

6.2.4 Systematic literature search for individual HTA aspects: search strategy and article selection

Including all study designs meant that the iterative procedure recommended by Linde (see ◘ Fig. 6.2) was extended. All reviews available for the respective complementary medical speciality were taken into account (as suggested). As this was not considered sufficient for a conclusive evaluation further informative material was assessed.

In addition, a representative indication (domain) was chosen for investigating the 'effectiveness/efficacy' aspect. All clinical study designs were accepted for the evaluation of the domain.

Selection of studies on effectiveness/efficacy – reviews
The databases for homeopathy literature generated according to the search strategy mentioned (Reference Manager Version 10) were screened with the terms 'systematic review' and 'meta-

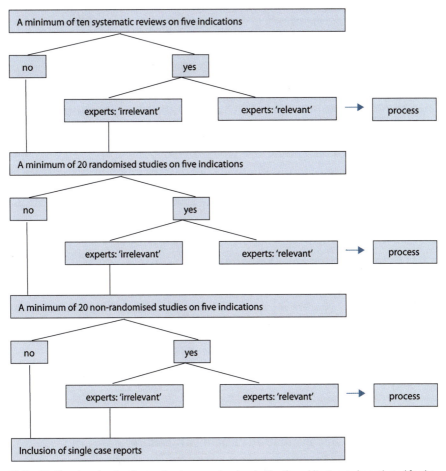

◘ **Fig. 6.2** Flowchart showing the step-by-step procedure in selecting the publications to be evaluated for the HTA (source: commission documents, K. Linde)

analysis' so that, on the basis of title lists and abstracts, studies that were irrelevant to the research question could be excluded. For the period leading up to 2000 the survey by Linde et al. (2001) was used as a basis.

Selection of studies on effectiveness/efficacy – domains (particular indications)
Depending on the domains chosen (for homeopathy they were 'upper respiratory tract infections' URTI) other specific search terms (for detailed list see below) were entered in the HTA databases and those accessible online (see ◘ Table 6.1).

Safety
Apart from a general search in the databases mentioned, the online database Toxline was screened using specialist search terms (homeopath*, homeopath*), partly in combination with side effects.

Health economy and demand
Next to the general search described in the previous paragraph various databases were also specially screened for aspects of 'health economy' and 'demand'.

Search strategy:
Name of medical speciality (homeopathy) was given in combination with key words ('health economics', 'costs') and extended by the term 'Switzerland' for search results specific to this country.

**Non-systematic literature search for introduction to the speciality
and pre-clinical effectiveness**
For the chapters that introduce homeopathy as a medical speciality, including the overview of pre-clinical research, no special search of the electronic databases took place. The material made available by the relevant experts was considered to be sufficient (mainly K. v. Ammon, S. Baumgartner, P. Mattmann and M. Righetti).

6.3   Data Extraction and Evaluation

Questionnaires were set up as data extraction and evaluation tools for the articles on the themes of 'effectiveness/efficacy', 'safety' and 'demand' (see Appendix). They corresponded in content and structure to the conventionally published questionnaires and forms (Chalmers et al. 1981, Jadad et al. 1996, Kleijnen et al. 2001; Busse et al. 'ECHTA' 2001; DAHTA/DIMDI 2004; Cochrane Coll. Handbook 2001) and to the Wein (2002) survey.

In addition, aspects of external validity relevant to the evaluation according to the PEK (Heusser 2001) and aspects specific to the individual complementary medical approaches were developed in collaboration with experts of the respective specialities.

6.3.1   Extraction and evaluation of data / procedure

Each full-text article for clinical trials was checked by two reviewers, those for systematic reviews and meta-analyses by at least one reviewer each. The relevant data were then extracted and evaluated using a questionnaire. Following the completion of the review, all data were compared and checked for consistency. Evaluation discrepancies were discussed, and a uniform set of data for PEK was drawn up for each article. There were no discrepancies that could not be resolved. The data sets formed the basis for further descriptive summaries.

6.3.2 Extraction and evaluation of data

Depending on the study design and the respective research question there were three **data extraction forms:**
- Review/meta-analysis
- Clinical trial
- Use of CAM ('demand') and costs

For single case analyses the questionnaire for clinical trials was used as a basis.

For further information regarding requirements and development and for questionnaire samples see Appendix.

Structure of data extraction form
The data extraction form is divided into three levels (see ◻ Fig. 6.3):

1. Description
For data extraction the published data and contents were assessed for each article based on a standardized procedure.

2. Internal validity
Based on the data extraction, potential bias factors were identified that might distort the study's internal validity.

3. External validity
The same categories of bias factors that were used for the evaluation of internal validity were also employed to evaluate external validity. In this context, the relevance and transferability of each publication to the PEK project and to Switzerland in particular were evaluated.

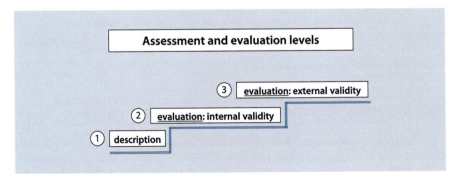

◻ **Fig. 6.3** Assessment and evaluation levels of the questionnaire

Content and structure of the data extraction (DE) forms (see also Appendix)

DE forms 'reviews/meta-analyses'
1. General information (bibliographical references, source, language, reviewer)
2. Background: research question and context (if applicable including intervention and indication; estimation of the question's internal and external validity)
3. Methodical aspects and information capture (data sources, inclusion and exclusion criteria, estimation of the internal and external validity of design)
4. Information synthesis (meta-analysis or other quantitative procedures, qualitative information synthesis)
5. Methods and results (answer to research question)
6. Current status and technology of HTA/ reviews; transferability of international/foreign results and conclusions (external validity)
7. Evaluation/recommendation (author's and reviewer's conclusion concerning effectiveness, if possible also safety and cost-effectiveness).

For systematic reviews a total of 76 individual aspects were assessed.

DE forms 'clinical trials'
1. General information (bibliographical references, source, language, reviewer)
2. Research question
3. Population/patient
4. Study design/methods
5. Intervention
6. Questions specific to homeopathy
7. Outcome and results
8. Statistics (analyses)
9. Evaluation/recommendation

A total of 98 individual aspects were assessed.

DE forms 'use/appropriateness/costs'
1. General information (bibliographical references, source, language, reviewer)
2. Background: research question and context
3. Study design
4. Results: frequency of CAM use, reasons for using CAM, health economics data
5. Evaluation/ recommendation

A total of 36 individual aspects were assessed.

6.3.3 Evaluation categories

The evaluation of publications for the present HTA followed the published, habitually used criteria for the evaluation of internal and external validity (Cochrane Coll. Handbook 2001, BSV Handbuch 2000, Heusser 1999, DIMDI 2004, Kleijnen et al. 2001) and the quality criteria set out by Wein (2002).

Evaluation of individual studies on three levels:
As shown above, data identification and evaluation took place on three levels:

1. **Description / documentation:** A documentation was rated 'good' if all aspects necessary for the assessment of internal and external validity were shown in the article. If the documentation is considered 'poor' the bias factors that result in distortion and reduced validity cannot be assessed.
2. **Internal validity:** The internal validity is the extent to which a study, by design or implementation, is able to avoid systematic errors. Evaluation took place under consideration of possible bias factors. For a more detailed description see Chap. 5. The evidence grades were listed together with the study description.
3. **External validity:** External validity means the validity of studies or study results transferred to a wider context: in the case of the PEK this is the transferability of results from other contexts to the situation in Switzerland.

The transferability of study results can change over time and is therefore a variable that needs to be evaluated within the given context.

Based on the data extracted, the reviewer assessed the internal and external validity (documentation level). An overall score was not established because individual factors such as randomisation, blinding, representativeness of the population etc. can carry different weight depending on the research question. Statements were then made, wherever possible, on how and to what extent the study result might be distorted. For the assessment and evaluation of these bias factors see the data extraction forms in the Appendix.

The procedure as used here is an extension of the commonly used evidence and validity evaluation. The reasons for this extension are described in detail in Chap. 5.

6.4 Data Synthesis

First, the data extracted from studies concerning a domain were described with their characteristics and key statements. Key characteristics, safety information and evaluations of internal and external validity were then tabulated.

For the description and evaluation of the studies included, research questions (indications), study design and methods (RCT, placebo control, blinding, baseline comparability, lost to follow-up), considerations of external validity (such as treatment determination according to the homeopathic similarity rule, the weight of symptoms, confounding factors), outcome parameters (clinical parameters, surrogate parameters, quality of life, costs etc.) were compared. Unexpected adverse events (UAE) that were described were also assessed.

The outcome synthesis was set out in a descriptive statistical form with thematic differentiation for which the study results (significance, trend or no difference in favour of or against the treatment) were listed and combined in a well-founded overall evaluation.

For the review articles the following criteria were used (adjusted from Glanville and Sowden 2001):

- What is the objective of the review?
- What **sources** were searched to identify primary studies? (What databases and other sources, what search strategies; were any restrictions used as to language, type of study etc.?)
- What were the **inclusion and exclusion criteria** and how were they applied?

- What criteria were used to assess the quality of primary studies and how were they applied (e.g. quality score according to Jadad or other **quality criteria**)?
- What **data/information** were extracted from the primary studies and how?
- How were the **data synthesized**? (How were differences between studies presented and interpreted? How were the results combined? Was it reasonable to combine them? What are the results of the review? Do the conclusions follow logically from the evidence established?)

Regarding the question of safety, the data on the frequency and severity of UAE were descriptively compiled, including the respective author's or reviewer's causality attribution, from studies that had been investigated with regard to 'effectiveness/efficacy' and also from studies that had been specifically identified under the heading of 'safety'.

The data on economy were tabulated and individually discussed and evaluated.

The concluding answer to the research question was developed out of the evaluations of the individual parts and well substantiated.

6.5   Publications

6.5.1   Database research 'Homeopathy'

Homeopathy: general search
- Time frame for search: 14 May–20 June 2003
- Search strategy for homeopathy in general (depending on database with truncation and wildcards as in hom?eopath#.af.)
- Results according to database (see ▢ Table 6.2)
- Generation of own 'homeopathy' database

▢ **Table 6.2** Number of articles found when entering the general search term 'homeopathy' into various databases

Database	Number of hits	Database	Number of hits
AMED	11234	Health Managem.	136
Embase	2409	PsycInfo	120
Medline	2272	Current Contents	97
Mantis	1603	Dissertation Abstr.	68
Cinahl	1518	Psyndex	59
Biosis	921	Premedline	52
Pascal	885	SIGLE	43
Pharmac. News	552	Soc. Science	28
Scrip & Scrip plus	363	MLA	26
EBMR	356	Philosoph. Index	11
Newspaper	242	Econlit	3

Table 6.3 Search for studies and case studies in the homeopathy database (electronic keyword search)

Search for	Number of hits
randomized, controlled study	133
clinical study	296
review, meta-analysis	393
meta-analysis only	51
cohort study	1
case study	59

For distribution according to study types (search terms entered into own database) see
◻ Table 6.3.
— Search in 'homeopathy' database (in Reference Manager 10) for randomized studies.
Search instruction RCT in 'abstract' yielded   16 articles
Search instruction randomized yielded   103 articles
Search instruction randomized yielded   293 articles with clear overlaps

From the list of titles (107 evaluable titles in all) a rough outline of the indications treated was
established (see ◻ Table 6.4).

Table 6.4 Proportional incidence of indications investigated in randomized studies on homeopathy

Indication	% of hom. RCTs
musculo-skeletal system/connective tissue (mainly rheumatoid arthritis)	18
urogenital system (incl. infertility and premenstrual complaints)	14
respiratory system (incl. asthma)	13
blood, immune system (incl. allergies, atopies)	12
nervous system (incl. headache)	8
skin and subcutis (incl. warts)	7
infections (incl. HIV, malaria)	5
digestive system	5
external causes (traumas, poisoning; insect bite, wound healing after surgery)	5
psychological and behavioural disorders	3
ear and mastoid process	3
other (altitude sickness, marathon)	3
metabolism (endocrine, nutrition)	2
▼	

Table 6.4 (continued)

Indication	% of hom. RCTs
pregnancy, birth and childbed	2
external causes of diseases	1
neoplasia	0
eye and ocular adnexa	0
circulary system	0
perinatal period	0
congenital malformations	0
abnormal clinical and laboratory findings	0
Total	100%

6

6.5.2 Special search: URTI (Upper Respiratory Tract Infection)

The search for articles (clinical studies and single case studies) for the chosen indication URTI was performed in two databases:

1. Search in general homeopathy file (see Sect. 6.5.); search terms: upper respiratory tract infection, laryngitis, tracheobronchitis, angina, otitis media, throat pain, rhinitis, rhinopharyngitis, glue ear, sinusitis, tracheitis, pharyngitis, tonsillitis, amygdalitis: 34 articles found altogether.
2. Special additional search in the online databases; the following databases were screened for articles on the selected indication 'URTI': Econlit, EMBASE, Pre-MEDLINE, MEDLINE Daily Update, MEDLINE.

Search strategy:

 1 hom?opath$.af. (4817)
 2 upper respiratory tract infection.af. (4775)
 3 laryngitis.af. (3615)
 4 tracheobronchitis.mp[mp=hw, ab, ti, ct, sh, tn, ot, dm, mf, rw] (625)
 5 angina.af. (72772)
 6 throat pain.af. (219)
 7 otitis media.af. (27300)
 8 rhinitis.af. (26253)
 9 rhinopharyngitis.af. (424)
10 glue ear.af. (385)
11 sinusitis.af. (20199)
12 tracheitis.af. (1599)
13 pharyngitis.af. (10137)
14 tonsillitis.af. (105)
15 amygdalitis.af. (27)

16 1 and 2 (19)
17 1 and 3 (7)
18 1 and 4 (0)
19 1 and 5 (18)
20 1 and 6 (0)
21 1 and 7 (36)
22 1 and 8 (59)
23 1 and 9 (0)
24 1 and 10 (3)
25 1 and 11 (22)
26 1 and 12
27 1 and 13 (9)
28 1 and 14 (0)
29 1 and 15 (0)
30 from 16 keep 1–10 (10)
31 from 16 keep 1–19 (19)

The result (after elimination of duplicates) was an overall file of 290 articles for URTI in which further search steps were carried out.

3. The most comprehensive compilation of clinical studies on homeopathy was done by Wein (2002), but his references regarding URTI could be considered only in part (due to differing inclusion criteria etc.).

4. Selection of titles from the URTI file:
   Based on the titles and abstracts, 41 studies were selected. Further research resulted in the exclusion of nine more studies. Three studies were not available as full text, so that the ultimate number of suitable studies was 29.

6.5.3 Safety

The database Toxline, which is specially designed for side effects and poisonings, was searched by entering the terms: homeopath* OR homeopath* and CAM. Homeopathy produced ca. 130 hits, all of which had already been retrieved from the databases described before and were not particularly relevant. More articles were located via bibliographic references and expert contacts.

6.5.4 Cost-effectiveness

Apart from the general search described in the preceding section, the various databases were also specially screened for the aspects 'health economics' and 'use'.

Search strategy:
Names of specialities (homeopathy, phytotherapy, TCM, neural therapy) were entered in combination with key words ('health economics', 'costs') and coupled with the term 'Switzerland' to obtain specific results for that country.

For the number of titles found in each database see ▢ Tables 6.5 and 6.6.

Table 6.5 Search 'health economics and CAM'

Cost effectiveness (detailed search see*)	health economic$.af.	economic$.af.	complemens med$.af.	alterns med$.af.	CAM.af.	CDSR, ACP Journal Club, DARE, CCTR	AMED	CINAHL	Current Contents/ Clinical Medicine	Dissertation Abstracts	Econlit	EMBASE	Mantis	Pre-MEDLINE, MEDLINE	Newspaper Abstracts	Pharmaceutical and Healthcare Industry News
×						12347	2786	25855	5774	36897	48773	162371	2224	191594	213300	46882
	×					331	23	2547	201	138	957	98728	16	3540	209	849
		×				2709	1960	20308	1898	63842	365851	98,728	1630	109404	232180	14,398
			×			231	2738	1832	221	114	5	3672	297	4158	72	109
				×		275	915	4157	355	185	26	5902	1505	2668	928	159
					×	102	248	802	265	954	21	6774	1551	7716	1339	109
×			×			105	77	72	10	5	2	115	19	83	6	19
	×		×			11	1	7	0	0	0	10	0	4	0	1
		×	×			35	77	93	2	3	3	36	10	28	2	7
×				×		75	39	101	22	15	4	494	77	188	49	44
	×			×		10	0	13	0	0	0	28	2	6	1	2
		×		×		33	18	175	5	23	16	163	61	58	10	17
×					×	16	14	25	7	47	1	91	12	93	57	21
	×				×	5	0	0	0	1	0	1	0	0	0	0
		×			×	9	6	47	1	18	7	22	7	27	15	4

* COST OF REPRODUCTION/ or HOSPITAL COST/ or COST EFFECTIVENESS ANALYSIS/ or COST UTILITY ANALYSIS/ or ENERGY COST/ or HOSPITAL RUNNING COST/ or COST CONTROL/ or DRUG COST/ or COST BENEFIT ANALYSIS/ or COST MINIMIZATION ANALYSIS/ or COST/ or cost$.mp. or HEALTH CARE COST/ or COST OF ILLNESS/

☐ **Table 6.6** Search 'health economics and type of therapy'										
trad$ chinese medic$.af	hom?eopath$.af.	phytotherap$.af	anthroposoph$.af.	neural therap$ or Neuraltherap$).af	complemen$ med$.af.	altern$ med$.af.	(econom$ or cost$).af.	Econlit	EMBASE	Pre-MEDLINE, MEDLINE
x								0	1235	3571
	x							3	2420	2345
		x						0	5024	8078
			x					0	87	142
				x				0	89	60
					x			5	3683	4194
						x		26	5942	2722
							x	429364	248504	307777
x							x	0	20	25
	x						x	1	157	76
		x					x	0	106	161
			x				x	0	9	11
				x			x	0	3	5
					x		x	4	135	105
						x	x	18	584	235

The first viewing of titles (1976) showed that the chosen key words were not distinctive enough. A further hand search of the list resulted in a file of 920 titles.

Exclusion criteria:

— Duplicates
— Newspaper articles from other countries with unpromising titles
— Political and commercial information that was obviously not related to CAM
— Nursing
— Acupuncture
— Traditional medicine (Columbia, native American etc.)
— Diet
— Behavioural training
— Technical descriptions (CAD/CAM)
— Physiological therapies (chiropractic)
— Editorial/letter/congress more than 5 years old
— Incorrect, not verifiable bibliographical references
— Physiological therapies

Inclusion criteria:
- Primary data collection
- Contributions to discussions
- Articles specifically from or about Switzerland
- Information to be expected on:
  - the use of CAM ('demand')
  - quality of life
  - costs/effectiveness

Relevant articles were selected by hand for use in the HTA report from an overall file of 831 articles.

6.6   References

Bundesamt für Sozialversicherung der Schweiz (ed. now: Bundesamt für Gesundheit BAG) (1996 and 2002) Handbuch zur Standardisierung der medizinischen und wirtschaftlichen Bewertung medizinischer Leistungen. Bern

Busse R, Orvain J, Drummond M, Gurtner F, Jørgensen T, Jovell A, Malone J, Perleth M, Wild C (2001) Best practice in undertaking and reporting HTA. ECHTA Working Group 4 Final Report July 2001. available at: http://www.oeaw.ac.at/ita/ebene5/WG4_FinalReport_010719.pdf

Chalmers TC, Smith H jr, Blackburn B, Silverman B, Schroeder B, Reitman D, Ambroz A (1981) A method for assessing the quality of a randomized control trial. Control Clin Trials 2:31–49

The Cochrane Collaboration (2001) Cochrane Reviewers Handbook. Handbook 4.1.4.

Deutsche Agentur für Health Technology Assessment (DAHTA) beim Deutschen Institut für medizinische Information und Dokumentation (DIMDI) (2004) HTA: Vorgehensweise, Konzept und Inhalt. Available at: http://www dimdi de/de/hta/hta_dimdi/Konzept html.

Glanville J, Sowden A. Identification of the need for a review. In: Khan K, ter Riet G, Glanville J, Sowden A, Kleijnen J (eds) (2001) Undertaking systematic reviews of research on effectiveness. CRD Report Number 4 (2nd edn), York

Heusser P (1999) Probleme von Studiendesigns mit Randomisation, Verblindung und Placebogabe. Forschende Komplementärmedizin 6:89–102

Heusser P (2001) Criteria for assessing benefit with complementary medical methods. [in German]. Forschende Komplementärmedizin und Klassische Naturheilkunde 8:14–23

International Network of Agencies for Health Technology Assessments (INAHTA) (2001) A Checklist for Health Technology Assessment Reports. http://www.dimdi.de/de/hta/hta_dimdi/inahtachecklist.pdf

Jadad AR, Moore RA, Carroll D, Jenkinson C, Reynolds DJM, Gavaghan DJ, McQuy HJ (1996) Assessing the quality of reports of randomized clinical trials: is blinding necessary? Control Clin Trials 17:1–12

Linde K, Hondras M, Vickers A, ter Riet G, Melchart D (2001) Systematic reviews of complementary therapies – an annotated bibliography. Part 3: Homeopathy. BMC Complement Alternat Med 1:4

NHS Centre for Reviews and Dissemination, Kleijnen J et al. Undertaking systematic reviews of research on effectiveness. CRD Report No 4.CRD Publications. Available at: http://www.york.ac.uk/inst/crd/report4.htm

Wein C (2002) Qualitätsaspekte klinischer Studien zur Homöopathie. KVC, Essen

International Utilisation of Complementary Medical Approaches

René Gasser, Ursula Wolf, Martin Wolf, Klaus v. Ammon,
Gudrun Bornhöft, Stefanie Maxion-Bergemann

7.1   Introduction and Research Questions

What kinds of individuals or groups are using CAM (complementary alternative medicine) for which reasons, and how often? These questions are of much interest to health authorities, service providers, service guarantors, the economy and the public in general. This chapter describes studies published on these topics in Europe and beyond. Studies from Switzerland are examined in more detail in Chapter 8.

The studies were evaluated with the following questions in mind:

- Profile of CAM users: Is the use of CAM evenly distributed among all strata of the population or are there groups that use CAM to a greater extent?
- Frequency of use: How often does the population use CAM?
- Estimate of effectiveness and satisfaction: How do users rate the effectiveness and their satisfaction with CAM?
- Reasons for use: What reasons are given for the use of CAM?
- CAM use in relation to conventional medicine use: Is CAM used substitutively or additionally?

The compilation of publications serves to provide an overview without claiming completeness. A list of all excluded studies and the reasons for exclusion is available from the authors.

7.2   Methodology

How the data were collected is described in chapter 6. There are two types of data collection and data analysis (Atteslander 1993, Bortz 2004, Friedrichs 1980, Schnell et al. 2004, Wellhöfer 1997).

1. Collection and analysis of primary data
Interviews:
Interviewing is the most important tool when collecting primary data to find answers to the research questions. Different designs are available:
- Frequency of questioning:
  Interviews are usually conducted at one set point in time (cross-sectional design). If changes are to be monitored over a period of time, the same participants are interviewed again at a later point in time (longitudinal design).
- Assessment period:
  The question regarding the use of CAM can refer to the past (retrospective) or to the future (prospective). In the case of a retrospective survey the length of time measured can vary considerably. The present study mostly examined one-year prevalence (assessment of the last 12 months) and lifetime prevalence (assessment during the entire lifetime).
- Method of communication:
  Interviews were conducted face-to-face or over the phone. For the surveys, questionnaires were handed out to the participants who noted down their answers and returned the questionnaires to the study centre.
- Questioning techniques:
  Questioning can be standardized, partly standardized and non-standardized. Non-standardized surveys are unguided, freely executed explorations while standardized interviews are fully structured which means the order and phrasing of questions as well as the answer categories are preset (Wellhöfer 1997).

2. Analysis of secondary data

It is also possible to evaluate data from existing sources that were primarily used for other purposes, such as patient files or previous publications.

7.3 Results

7.3.1 Outline of studies used

At total of 52 studies which investigated CAM in general were used for the evaluation. They are listed in ◘ Table 7.1. The present chapter refers to these studies with the study number (SN) allocated to them in the table.

The studies are from nine countries: 30 (or about half) of them are from the United States. Of the remainder 15 are European (six from Germany, four from Britain, three from Sweden and one each from Slovenia and Italy), three from Canada, three from Australia and one from New Zealand.

The following kinds of studies were excluded: studies that were not concerned with at least one of the research questions set out above; studies that were not written in German or English; studies that were not concerned with at least one of the five complementary medical specialties relevant for the Swiss KVG health insurance programme (anthroposophic medicine, homeopathy, neural therapy, phytotherapy, traditional Chinese medicine).

Other international studies that investigated CAM use in connection with economic aspects are discussed in Chap. 12.

7.3.2 Study design

All but four (nos. 8, 26, 33, 36) studies were cross-sectional and collected data at only one point in time. Six different population groups were assessed by the studies. One essential difference was whether the studies were conducted with patients in a health-care institution or by a representative survey of the entire population in an area. The ratio was as follows: 18.5% adults without and 27.7% with specific indication; for a further 7.4% a subgroup with a specific indication was compared with other patients; 11.1% were young patients (children) with or without a specific indication and 29.6% belonged to the general population of a particular area. For 5.6% of the studies CAM therapists were interviewed.

A majority of 49 studies collected primary data. Six of these included additional secondary data in their analysis (nos. 2, 3, 12, 14, 25, 36). The following methods of questioning were used: with 20 (40.8%) of the studies the participants were sent a questionnaire, with 15 (30.6%) telephone interviews took place and with 14 (28.6%) interviewer and interviewee met face to face.

The results of the other studies (nos. 21, 32, 40) are based on secondary data.

The studies almost exclusively examined the past use of CAM; 47 of the 52 studies used only retrospective questions, four other studies (nos. 12, 28, 34, 47) combined retrospective and prospective questions to retrieve also information about the possible course of the CAM use; one study (no. 33) was prospective.

7

◼ Table 7.1 List of studies and their properties

SN	First author	Title	Year	Country
1	Al-Windi A	The relationship between age, gender, well-being and symptoms, and the use of pharmaceuticals, herbal medicines and self-care products in a Swedish municipality.	2000	Sweden
2	Anderson DL	Prevalence and patterns of alternative medication use in a University hospital outpatient clinic serving rheumatology and geriatric patients	2000	USA
3	Armishaw J	Use of complementary treatment by those hospitalized with acute illness	1999	New Zealand
4	Brown CM	The effects of health and treatment perceptions on the use of prescribed medication and home remedies among African-American and white American hypertensives	1996	USA
5	Davis MP	Use of complementary and alternative medicine by children in the United States	2003	USA
6	Dinehart SM	Use of alternative therapies by patients undergoing surgery for non-melanoma skin cancer	2002	USA
7	Drivdahl CE	The use of alternative health care by a family practice population	1998	USA
8	Eisenberg DM	Trends in alternative medicine use in the United States, 1990–1997: results of a follow-up national survey	1998	USA
9	Eisenberg DM	Unconventional medicine in the United States: prevalence, costs, and patterns of use	1993	USA
10	Elder NC	Use of alternative health care by family practice patients	1997	USA
11	Ernst E	The BBC survey of complementary medicine use in the UK	2000	GB
12	Fairfield KM	Patterns of use, expenditures, and perceived efficacy of complementary and alternative therapies in HIV-infected patients	1998	USA
13	Foster DF	Alternative medicine use in older Americans	2000	USA
14	Furler MD	Use of complementary and alternative medicine by HIV-infected outpatients in Ontario, Canada	2003	Canada
15 ▼	Giese L	A study of alternative health care use for gastro-intestinal disorders	2000	USA

Participants	Source of secondary data	Method of data collection	Method of questioning	Indication	n (r%)
population		retrospective	questionnaire	all	1312 (63)
patients (adults, specific indication)	patient files	retrospective	telephone interview	rheumato-logy and geriatric patients	176
patients (children, specific indication)	patient files	retrospective	interview	severe illness	251
population (adults)		retrospective	telephone interview	hyper-tension	300
population (children)		retrospective	interview	all	6262
patients (adults, specific indication)		retrospective	questionnaire	non-melanoma skin cancer	192 (58)
patients (adults, general)		retrospective	questionnaire	all	177(71)
population (adults)		retrospective, longitudinal	telephone interview	all	2055 (60, weighted)
population (adults)		retrospective	telephone interview	all	1539 (67)
patients (adults, general)		retrospective	questionnaire	all	113 (87)
population		retrospective	telephone interview	all	1204
patients (adults, specific indication)	patient files	combined (retro- + pro-spective)	telephone interview	HIV	180 (76)
population (older adults)		retrospective	telephone interview	all	311 (60)
patients (adults, specific indication)	patient files	retrospective	interview	HIV	208 (44)
patients (adults, specific indication)		retrospective	questionnaire	gastro-intestinal disorders	73

◘ Table 7.1 (continued)

SN	First author	Title	Year	Country
16	Gray CM	Complementary and alternative medicine use among health plan members. A cross-sectional survey	2002	USA
17	Haetzman M	Chronic pain and the use of conventional and alternative therapy	2003	GB
18	Haltenhof H	Evaluation and prevalence of CAM therapies – a survey among 793 physicians in general practice and hospitals	1995	Germany
19	Hanyu N	Utilization of complementary and alternative medicine by United States adults	2002	USA
20	Hayes KM	Alternative therapies and nurse practitioners: knowledge, professional experience, and personal use	2000	USA
21	Hentschel C	ICD-diagnoses in a naturopathic university policlinic	1996	Germany
22	Hsiao AF	Complementary and alternative medicine use and substitution for conventional therapy by HIV-infected patients	2003	USA
23	Kaboli P	Use of complementary and alternative medicine by older patients with arthritis: a population-based study	2001	USA
24	Kappauf H	Use of and attitudes held towards unconventional medicine by patients in a department of internal medicine/oncology and haematology.	2000	Germany
25	Kemper KJ	Consultations for holistic pediatric services for inpatients and outpatient oncology patients at a children‹s hospital	2001	USA
26	Kessler RC	Long-term trends in the use of complementary and alternative medical therapies in the United States	2001	USA
27	Kessler R	The use of complementary and alternative therapies to treat anxiety and depression in the United States	2001	USA
28	Kindermann A	Why do patients choose a TCM clinic?	1998	Germany
29	Langmead L	Use of complementary therapies by patients with IBD may indicate psychosocial distress	2002	GB
30	Lee MM	Complementary and alternative medicine use among men with prostate cancer in 4 ethnic populations	2002	USA

Participants	Source of secondary data	Method of data collection	Method of questioning	Indication	n (r%)
population (adults)		retrospective	questionnaire	all	4404 (86)
patients (adults, general)		retrospective	questionnaire	chronic pain	1608 (83)
physicians		not documented	questionnaire	all	1275 (62)
population (adults)		retrospective	direct interview	All	30801 (70)
physicians		retrospective	questionnaire	all	202 (73)
patients (adults, general)	patient files	retrospective		various	208
patients (adults, specific indication)		retrospective	interview	HIV	2466 (86 of baseline-population)
patients (adults, specific indication)		retrospective	telephone interview	arthritis	480 (62)
patients (adults, general and specific indication)		retrospective	direct interview	3 groups: all, cancer and out-patients	131 (98)
patients (children, general)	patient files	retrospective	questionnaire	oncology patients	70 (100)
population		retrospective longitudinal	telephone interview	all	2055 (60)
population (adults)		retrospective	telephone interview	anxiety, depression	2055 (60)
patients (adults, general)		retro- and prospective	interview	various conditions (mostly chronic)	94
patients (adults, general and specific indication)		retrospective	questionnaire	IBD	239 (98)
patients (adults, specific indication)		retrospective	telephone interview	oncology (prostate cancer)	543 (70 with 30 min. interview)

□ Table 7.1 (continued)

SN	First author	Title	Year	Country
31	Matthees BJ	Use of complementary therapies, adherence, and quality of life in lung transplant recipients	2001	USA
32	McFarland B	Complementary and alternative medicine use in Canada and the USA	2002	Canada/USA
33	Melchart D	Systematic clinical auditing in complementary medicine: rationale, concept, and a pilot study.	1997	Germany
34	Menniti-Ip-polito F	Use of unconventional medicine in children in Italy	2002	Italy
35	Messerer M	Socio-demographic and health behaviour factors among dietary supplement and natural remedy users	2001	Sweden
36	Messerer M	Use of dietary supplements and natural remedies increased dramatically during the 1990s	2001	Sweden
37	Norred C	Complementary and alternative medicine use by surgical patients	2002	USA
38	Palinkas L	The use of complementary and alternative medicine by primary care patients: a surf-net study	2000	USA
39	Pitetti R	Complementary and alternative medicine use in children	2001	USA
40	Premik M	Alternative medicine in Slovenia: some socio-medical views	1998	Slovenia
41	Rajendran PR	The use of alternative therapies by patients with Parkinson‹s disease	2001	USA
42	Schäfer T	Alternative medicine in allergies. Prevalence, patterns of use, and costs	2002	Germany
43	Sharples FM	NHS patients‹ perspective on complementary medicine: a survey.	2003	GB

7

Participants	Source of secondary data	Method of data collection	Method of questioning	Indication	n (r%)
patients (adults, specific indication)		retrospective	questionnaire	lung- or heart-lung transplants	99 (68)
patients (adults, general)	other data sources	retrospective		all	Canada: 70884 (83), USA: 16400 (78)
patients (adults, general) and physicians		prospective longitudinal	questionnaire	all	1597 (97% before, 84% 2 mos after, 78% 6 mos after, 70% 12 mos after treatment)
population (children)		retrospective	interview	all	70898
population		retrospective	interview	all	11422
population		retrospective longitudinal	interview	all	38594 (81)
patients (adults, specific indication)		retrospective	interview	surgical intervention (outpatient)	6852 (91)
patients (adults, general)		retrospective	interview	all	541 (89)
patients (children, general)		retrospective	questionnaire	all	525 (68)
physicians as well as patient population	two studies referred to in detail	retrospective	partly questionnaire, partly not documented	all	870 and 1650
patients (adults, specific indication)		retrospective	interview	Parkinson's disease	201 (91)
patients (adults, specific indication)		retrospective	telephone interview	allergies	351
patients in a homeopathic hospital		retrospective	questionnaire	all	499 (64)

7

■ **Table 7.1** (continued)

SN	First author	Title	Year	Country
44	Shenfield G	Survey of the use of complementary medicines and therapies in children with asthma	2002	Australia
45	Unützer J	Mental disorders and the use of alternative medicine: results from a national survey	2000	USA
46	Von Peter S	Survey on the use of complementary and alternative medicine among patients with headache syndromes	2002	USA
47	Wang Y	A pilot study of the use of alternative medicine in multiple sclerosis patients with special focus on acupuncture	1999	Canada
48	Wilkinson JM	High use of complementary therapies in a New South Wales rural community	2001	Australia
49	Wilkinson JM.	Complementary therapy use by nursing, pharmacy and biomedical science students	2001	Australia
50	Wolsko P	Patterns and perceptions of care for treatment of back and neck pain: results of a national survey	2003	USA
51	Yeh GY	Use of complementary and alternative medicine among persons with diabetes mellitus: results of a national survey	2002	USA
52	Yoon SL	Herbal products and conventional medicines used by community-residing older women	2001	USA

Abbreviations: *SN* study number; *n* number of respondents, *(r: %)* response rate, *HIV* human immuno-deficiency virus, *GB* Great Britain; *TCM* traditional Chinese medicine, *IBD* irritable bowel disease

7.3.3 CAM definitions

There is no generally valid definition of CAM (19) and the various studies define the term differently. Its meaning also changes over time. The 'Office of Alternative Medicine' of the US National Institutes of Health (NIH) held a methodology symposium in 1995 which arrived at the following definition: 'A broad domain of healing resources that encompass all health systems, modalities and practices, and their accompanying theories and beliefs, other than those intrinsic to the politically dominant health system of a particular society or culture in a given historical period. It includes all such products and ideas self-defined by their users as preventing

Participants	Source of secondary data	Method of data collection	Method of questioning	Indication	n (r%)
patients (children, specific indication)		retrospective	interview	asthma	children: 174 (93; parents: 331
population (adults, specific indication and other)		retrospective	telephone interview	mental health prob-lems	9585 (64)
patients (adults, specific indication)		retrospective	interview, partly direct, partly by phone	headaches	73
patients (adults, specific indication)		combined (retro- + prospective)	questionnaire	multiple sclerosis	848 (52)
population (adults)		retrospective	questionnaire	all	300 (31)
population (students)		retrospective	questionnaire	all	271 (72)
patients (adults, specific indication)		retrospective	telephone interview	back and neck pain	2055 (60, weighted)
population (adults, general; subgroup comparison: diabetes mellitus)		retrospective	telephone interview	diabetes mellitus	2055 (60, weighted)
population (adults, older women)		retrospective	questionnaire	various conditions (mostly chronic)	86 (21.5)

or treating illness or promoting health and well-being. Boundaries within complementary and alternative medicine and between complementary and alternative medicine and the domain of the dominant system are not always sharp or fixed' (Kelner et al., 2000, quoted from Dixon et al. 2003).

This implies that CAM definitions are specific to a culture and time period and depend on the prevailing mode of 'mainstream medicine'.

◘ Table 7.2 shows the different CAM definitions used in the studies. It is obvious that the different CAM definitions have to be taken into account when the studies are compared (e.g. for subgroup formation and analysis).

7

◼ **Table 7.2** CAM definitions in the studies used (grouped)

Study number	CAM definition	Operationalisation of CAM definition
6, 7, 8, 9, 12, 13, 15, 16, 22, 23, 26, 31, 38, 46, 49, 50, 51	'medical interventions, not taught widely at US medical schools or generally available at US hospitals' (according to Eisenberg 1993)	list of therapies/methods (number of therapies/methods asked about varies between 12 and 49)
14	'any treatment not commonly provided by physicians or medical practitioners, and used in conjunction with or in place of standard medical treatments' (adjusted from Eisenberg 1993)	verbal explanation of adjacent definition
44, 45	respondents' own definition	respondents' own definition (with examples given in some cases)
2	'any product, including herbal remedies, vitamins, minerals and natural products, that may be purchased without a prescription at a health food store, pharmacy or supermarket, or from alternative medicine magazines or catalogues for the purpose of self-treatment'	asked about use according to adjacent definition
10	traditional medicine: 'care received from their physician or doctor of osteopathy and any treatments he or she recommends or prescribes, including physical therapy, medications, or counselling'; CAM: 'seeing a non-traditional or alternative professional or using home remedies (including chiropractic, acupuncture, massage therapy, naturopathy, herbs and others)'	list of included therapies/ methods
20	'Office of Alternative Medicine' definition and list	list of 30 therapies/methods
5	'the integration of non-allopathic methods into preventive or acute health care'	list of 12 therapies/methods
19	'health care practices that are not an integral part of conventional medicine' (according to the National Institutes of Health)	list of 13 therapies/methods
41	standardized explanation of each therapy	list of 17 therapies/methods
24	providers, methods and modes of diagnostics, treatment and/or prevention, for which, without sound evidence, specificity, sensitivity and/or therapeutic efficacy is commonly claimed in respect to a definite medical problem	asked about use in accordance with adjacent definition
42	distinct therapeutic procedures **not** including herbs, food supplements, home remedies or minor adjuvant measures	respondents' answers according to adjacent definition
35, 36	without definition	vitamins/strengthening and natural remedies
3, 4, 11, 17, 18, 27, 29, 30, 32, 34, 39, 40, 47, 48	without definition	no answers or list of therapies/ methods (number of therapies/methods asked about varies between 4 and 21)
1, 21, 25, 28, 33, 37, 43, 52	definition of CAM areas	Asked about use of respective sub-areas

7.3.4 Profile of CAM users

Many studies focus on the comparison of patients using CAM therapies with those using conventional medical methods. These studies have different results, but some trends are noticeable:

- Age: members of the middle age segment (between 30 and 50 years of age) use CAM most often or, put differently, CAM users are on average younger than non-CAM users (8, 9, 11, 16, 17, 19, 29, 30, 32, 37, 40, 41, 42, 45, 52).
- Gender: The results of 23 studies indicate that women use CAM therapies more often than men (1, 5, 6, 7, 8, 11, 14, 16, 17, 19, 23, 24, 29, 31, 35, 37, 39, 40, 45, 48, 50).
- Education: In 17 studies, respondents with a higher level of education specified significantly more often that they were using CAM (8, 9, 14, 16, 19, 22, 30, 31, 32, 34, 35, 37, 38, 40, 41, 42, 45).
- Income: CAM users tend to belong to a higher income bracket than non-users (5, 8, 9, 11, 41).

In addition to the trends mentioned above, there are also studies which found no (significant) differences between users and non-users of CAM for specific properties (1, 3, 4, 7, 10, 12, 13, 27, 39). With some of these studies the number of interviewees was too small for a significant difference to be established (3, 4, 7, 10, 12). In one study (35) CAM was used primarily by older people.

7.3.5 Frequency of CAM use

The majority of studies (25 of the 48 that are relevant to this question) assessed the use of CAM therapies over the preceding 12 months (1-year prevalence). Two of them (3, 23) also assessed the lifetime prevalence. Six further studies assessed only the lifetime prevalence of CAM use. Other time intervals observed were: present use of CAM therapies (three studies), use over the past fortnight (one study), 30 days (one study), 2 years (one study) and 3 years (one study) and one study which specified the time as '2 weeks leading up to surgery'. With another eight studies the period of use was not mentioned in the text.

Some studies investigated several time frames and therefore appear more than once in the table.

- One-year prevalence, studies without specific indication: the prevalence in the 13 studies without specific indication that assessed the use of CAM in the previous year was between 1.6% and 78% (median 30.4%). A study of children showed the lowest use. The lowest use in a study of adults was 5%.

Apart from country-specific preferences, the reasons for the wide discrepancies in the use of CAM therapies are probably due to differing CAM definitions and study designs (method and time of interview, observation period, population).

The study with the highest prevalence was conducted among health-care professionals. ◻ Table 7.1 contains more details on the studies and their design. With regard to the 1-year prevalence data, it should be considered that a part of the population interviewed was not ill in that year and therefore needed no treatment, which means they are not included in the result. The 1-year prevalence data therefore tend to be too low.

7

▣ Table 7.3 Outline: frequency of CAM use

SN	Frequency of use	Period of time	Indication
1-year prevalence, all disorders			
1	31.8% (263 of 827) phytotherapy	in previous year	all disorders
5	1.6% (101 of 6262)	in previous year	all disorders
7	28.2% (50 of 177)	in previous year	all disorders
8	42.1% (865 of 2055); comparison with a study of 1990 showed an increase for 15 of 16 therapies; 46.3% of CAM users consulted a CAM therapist.	in previous year	all disorders
9	34% (523 of 1539); of these, 36% of CAM users consulted a CAM therapist.	in previous year	all disorders
11	20% (254 of 1204), upward trend	in previous year	all disorders
13	30 % (93 of 311) of over 65-year-olds and 46% (800 of 1738) of under 65-year-olds	in previous year	all disorders
16	42% (1850 of 4404)	in previous year	all disorders
19	28.9% (8902 of 30,801)	in previous year	all disorders
32	Canada: 16% (11,400 of 70,884), USA: 5% (862 of 16,400)	in previous year	all disorders
38	21% (116 of 541)	in previous year	all disorders
48	70.3% (211 of 300), 62.7% (188 of 300) consulted a CAM therapist; TCM: 6%	in previous year	all disorders
49	77.9% (211 of 271), 56.3% (152 of 271) consulted a CAM therapist; TCM: 6%	in previous year	all disorders
1-year prevalence, specific indications			
2	66% (117 of 176)	in previous year	rheumatology and geriatric patients
3	18% (44 of 251)	in previous year	severe illness
12	67.8% (122 of 180) use of phytotherapeutics, vitamins or nutritional supplements; 15% (81 of 180) consulted a CAM therapist; TCM: 10.6%	in previous year	HIV
17	18.9% (94 of 840) consulted a CAM therapist; 15.7% (78 of 840) used CAM products	in previous year	chronic pain
23	16% (79 of 480), 57% (273 of 480) consulted CAM therapists	in previous year	arthritis
27	56.7% (110 of 193) of respondents with anxiety syndrome and 53.6% (79 of 148) of respondents with depression, 20% of respondents with anxiety syndrome and 19.3% of respondents with depression consulted a CAM therapist	in previous year	anxiety, depression
▼			

◘ **Table 7.3** (continued)

SN	Frequency of use	Period of time	Indication
30	30.2% (208 of 690)	in previous year	prostate cancer
31	88% (88 of 99) used at least one CAM therapy, 70.1% (69 of 99) used at least two CAM therapies	in previous year	lung or heart-lung transplantation
45	16.5% not weighted (14.4% weighted), of whom 45.6% consulted a CAM therapist	in previous year	mental health problems
50	29% (596 of 2055), 12% (246 of 2055) consulted a CAM therapist	in previous year	back and neck pain
51	diabetics: 57% (54 of 95); non-diabetics: 54.5% (1068 of 1960)	in previous year	diabetes mellitus
52	45.3% (39 of 86)	in previous year	(mostly) chronic disorders
lifetime prevalence			
20	63.4% (128 of 202)	lifetime	all disorders
26	67.6%, prevalence is increasing and is higher among younger people	lifetime	all disorders
3	29% (72 of 251)	lifetime	severe illness
23	66% (318 of 480), 28% (133 of 480) saw CAM therapists	lifetime	arthritis
28	58.6% had seen a CAM practitioner at least once; 73.7% had seen a non-medical practitioner at least once	lifetime	(mostly) chronic complaints
29	26% (62 of 239); TCM (herbs only): 8%	lifetime	inflammatory bowel diseases
41	40% (81 of 201), 26% (21 of 81) of whom said they use two CAM therapies, 33% (27 of 81) more than 2 und 12% (10 of 81) more than 5	lifetime	Parkinson's disease
44	51.7% (90 of 174) resp. 62.8% (91 of 145) of the therapies are used daily	lifetime (children)	asthma
other time frames, in order of length			
37	67% (4591 of 6 852), with several CAM methods being used simultaneously the authors state that 49% of the respondents used between two and 83 remedies (e.g. vitamins) and methods	2 weeks prior to surgery	outpatient surgery
6	18.8% (36 of 192)	present use	skin cancer (non- melanoma)
14	77% (160 of 208), 51% of whom relative to HIV	present use	HIV
24 ▼	24% (31 of 128) patients in general, 32% (26 of 81) cancer patients, 9% (3 of 34) chronic and 10% (1 of 10) acute benign illness	present use	cancer and other illness

□ Table 7.3 (continued)

SN	Frequency of use	Period of time	Indication
35, 36	nutritional supplements: 1996–97: 33.3% women and 22.2% men 1988–89: 23.9% women and 14.3% men 1980–81: 22.9% women and 13.4% men naturopathic medicines: 1996–97: 13.7% women and 7.3% men 1988–89: 11.0% women and 4.8% men 1980–81: 5.7% women and 2.2% men	past fortnight	all disorders
4	22% (66 of 300)	past month (30 days)	hypertension
15	43% (32 of 73)	past 2 years	gastrointestinal disorders
34	15.6%, compared with earlier studies, increasing prevalence	past 3 years	all disorders
10	50% (57 of 113);	not stated	all disorders
18	38.6% of physicians use one of 18 CAM methods listed; 62.5% of physicians are in favour of CAM.	not stated (less relevant here because interviewees were physicians)	all disorders
22	52.5% (115,400 of 219,700 – weighted according to place and other socio-demographic data based on 2466 interviewees!)	not stated	HIV
39	10.9% (57 of 525) of the children treated with CAM therapies, 31.4% of parents use CAM	not stated	all disorders
40	57.3% of 870 Slovenian interviewees and 37% of 1650 patients asked used CAM	not stated	all disorders
42	26.5% of 351, 64% of which prescribed by a physician and 22.6% with the physician's support	not stated (presumably lifetime prevalence)	allergies
46	84% (61 of 73)	not stated	headaches
47	67% (566 of 848)	not stated	multiple sclerosis

SN study number, *TCM* percentage of TCM use (if stated), *HIV* human immunodeficiency virus

- Lifetime prevalence, studies without specific indication: two studies (20, 26) that investigated the lifetime prevalence of CAM use did not restrict the indication. They documented that a majority of the population use CAM (63.4% resp. 67.6%). The first population investigated consisted of trainee nurses who had come across CAM in their training. The second higher prevalence was found in a representative survey among the US population.
  As lifetime prevalence assesses a much longer period of time than 1-year prevalence it is naturally higher.
- No time period specified: four studies (10, 18, 39, 40) without restriction of indication specified no time period. The prevalence of CAM usage shown was 50%, 38.6%, 31% and 57.3%. In the case of study no. 18 it has to be taken into account that the respondents were physicians, 38.6% of whom were themselves CAM prescribers and 62.5% of whom were in favour of CAM.

In summary, it can be said that an average 1-year prevalence of ca. 33% and a lifetime prevalence of ca. 66% was established for the use of CAM.

All studies that investigated the prevalence over a longer period of time found a strong increase in the use of CAM over the years (34, 35, 36).

Studies with specific indications: the range of indications covered is another aspect that needs special consideration. Evaluation was carried out partly using subgroups and analysis. Twenty-one of the 48 studies did not restrict themselves to a specific indication but investigated the general use of CAM in the population. The remaining 27 studies investigated specially defined indications.

- HIV: Three studies (12, 14, 22) looked at the prevalence of CAM use among HIV patients. These studies are not fully comparable, as each investigated a different time frame. For all three of them the percentage of CAM therapy users was very high; 63% and 77% of respondents said they had used CAM therapies or were still using them.
- Pain: Three studies (46, 17, 50) each investigated a particular kind of pain (headache, chronic pain, back and neck pain). A very high prevalence of use was reported for the headache syndrome (84%), although it is not clear to what time period this result relates. The results of the two other studies are considerably lower: 18.9% and 12% (consultation of a CAM therapist) and 15.7% and 29% (use of CAM products).
- Other indications: the prevalence of CAM therapy use for all other indications varies between 14.4% (mental health problems) and 88% (patients who received a lung or heart/lung transplant).
  In restriction, it must be added that not all studies differentiated between specific CAM use for a particular indication such as diabetes mellitus or HIV infection and general CAM use (e.g. HIV patient takes chamomile tea for stomach complaints).

7.3.6 Estimation of satisfaction with CAM and CAM effectiveness

Fifteen of the studies examined the satisfaction with CAM expressed by the respondents and the subjective effectiveness of the CAM therapies.

Table 7.4 shows patient satisfaction and subjective effectiveness in the individual studies.

The different studies show a high satisfaction rate with CAM therapies, with 46% and 62% (median 49.3%) of respondents indicating that they were 'quite satisfied' to 'very satisfied' with the CAM therapies or classifying the treatment received as 'very helpful'.

▪ Table 7.4 Estimated satisfaction with CAM and effectiveness of CAM

SN	Satisfaction with therapy	Effectiveness of therapy
7	49% were 'satisfied' to 'very satisfied'	82% reported at least slight improvement of their condition (40% of them reported major improvement and 8% said they were cured)
24	62% of patients feel better mentally with CAM	60% of patients reported mild to noticeable improvement with CAM
29	46% (with irritable bowel disease) or 53% (patients without IBD) were 'quite satisfied' to 'very satisfied'	
31		68.9% 'quite effective' or 'moderately effective'; 15% 'very effective'; 15% 'little effective' to 'no effect at all'.
33		70% improvement according to physician; significant improvement according to patients
39	28.6% of parents were 'very satisfied' with the results; 12% of parents were 'not at all satisfied' with the results	73.1% of parents reported an improvement in their child's condition
40		95% reported successful (49%) or partly successful (46%) treatment
42		82.4% consider CAM treatment to be effective with 28.6% of them stating very good and 53.8% quite good effectiveness; 38% of patients thought CAM to be better than conventional medicine, another 23.9% considered it equally good. Only 22.8% reported lower effectiveness. A quarter of patients did not require any other treatment due to CAM.
43		81.4% of patients reported improvement with 67% experiencing strong to medium and 19.5% slight improvement.
45	20.3% of CAM users were not satisfied with their treatment.	
46		in 60% of cases an improvement of the symptoms was reported
47		Acupuncture only: 64% of respondents reported strong improvement of their condition
50	48% of therapies were rated 'very helpful'	
51	60.6% experienced the treatment used as 'very helpful'	
52		47.9% experienced the treatment used as 'slightly effective' to 'very effective'.

SN study number

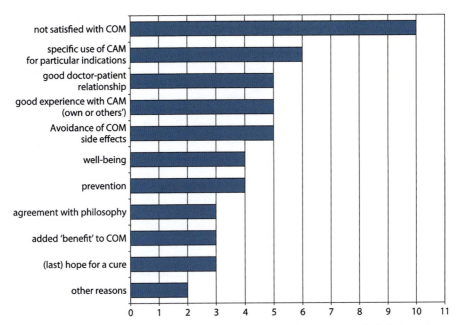

Fig. 7.1 Reasons for using CAM with number of times stated (repeated statements possible). *CAM* complementary alternative medicine, *COM* conventional (mainstream) medicine

The percentages are even higher for the effectiveness of CAM therapies: between 60% and 95% (median 82%) of respondents found that their condition had improved as a result of the therapy.

In summary, satisfaction with CAM was high and the estimated effectiveness of CAM very high.

7.3.7 Reasons for using CAM

Some of the studies examined the reasons for using CAM (nos. 2, 6, 10, 11, 12, 24, 25, 31, 34, 38, 39, 42, 43, 44 and 52).

In some studies the reasons for not using CAM were also mentioned: no health insurance, (assumed) lack of scientific evidence, lack of trust in the effectiveness of CAM treatment and general satisfaction with conventional medicine.

■ Fig. 7.1 shows the reasons for using CAM therapies.

The most frequently stated reason is dissatisfaction with conventional medicine, followed by specific use for a particular indication. An (assumed) good physician-patient relationship as well as the avoidance of the side effects of conventional medicine were also considered important. Other reasons stated by respondents were the higher amount of medical attention and longer treatment times with CAM therapists and the holistic philosophy underlying the CAM therapies.

7.3.8 Use of CAM compared with conventional medicine

In some studies CAM and conventional medicine were used simultaneously (8, 9, 18, 24, 25, 33, 45, 52). A few studies specified the use of CAM and COM in more detail (7, 22, 42, 43). In study no. 42 a quarter of the respondents who used CAM were able to do without conventional medical treatment altogether. Study no. 7 showed that in 66% of cases CAM was used parallel to conventional treatment, in 16% instead of, and in another 18% whenever COM had not helped. In study no. 22, 3% used CAM instead of conventional treatment. Study no. 43 reported a reduction of COM medicines as a result of the CAM therapy: 29% of patients needed no COM medication, 32% were able to reduce their COM medication, 33% maintained the same COM dosage and 6% had to increase it.

In a study among physicians (no. 18), the interviewees saw CAM as complementary to COM; a third favoured CAM over conventional treatment.

7.4 Discussion

There are numerous international studies covering various aspects of CAM use. Studies relating to the situation in Switzerland are dealt with in Chap. 8.

For the interpretation of the study results the following aspects need to be considered: (a) The definitions of CAM varied, also in width, and were often not very specific. (b) The time period to which the study questions related varied (1-year prevalence, lifetime prevalence or not defined). (c) The user groups questioned varied between 'average population' to a highly selected patient population with a specific indication in a specialist clinic or practice. (d) Depending on the studies' country of origin different CAM methods were investigated.

The factors mentioned led to a wide variability in study results and require subgroup formation and analysis to ensure adequate interpretation.

As most studies examined the use of CAM in general with only a few specifying particular CAM specialities, conclusions also refer to CAM in general rather than to individual CAM approaches.

The profile of CAM users compared with that of pure COM users reveals different trends: CAM users belong to the middle age segment (between 30 and 50 years old) and to a higher income bracket; they tend to be women and have a higher level of education. There are, however, also studies that do not confirm these tendencies. Influencing factors are, besides study design and population examined, differences between countries and the availability of individual CAM methods.

The prevalence of CAM use differs from one study to the next. In general, it was established that the use of CAM therapies was very high, with a 1-year prevalence of one third and a lifetime prevalence of two thirds of respondents. In recent years the use of CAM has also been rising noticeably.

Effectiveness was rated very high by users. Approximately half of the respondents were satisfied with the therapy. More than 80% gave a positive answer when asked if their condition had improved due to the therapy.

Different reasons were given for the use of CAM therapies: conventional treatments that had remained unsuccessful, as supplement and prophylaxis, additional benefit to conventional medicine as well as avoidance and reduction of the disadvantages of conventional medical treatment. Expectations from CAM treatment ranged from the alleviation of existing symptoms to the achievement of a cure. Other reasons for CAM use were, besides the wish to avoid the side effects of conventional medicine, the greater attention and longer treatment times devoted to patients by CAM therapists and the holistic views underlying the CAM therapies.

On the basis of the studies, the question of whether CAM is used as a substitute for conventional treatment (full or part substitution) or in addition to it (additional simultaneous or consecutive use) cannot be conclusively answered. Only few studies addressed this issue. Most studies reported the simultaneous use of CAM and conventional medicine. Some indicate simultaneous and substitutive usage. What makes the evaluation more difficult is that the terms are not clearly defined in the individual studies and a combination must be assumed. It is difficult to allocate genuine 'complementary' effects such as improved quality of life, the lowering of side effects or reduction of conventional medicines to the categories 'additive' or 'substitutive'. Future studies should take this important aspect into more serious consideration.

How do the results of the present HTA compare with those of two other surveys (Ernst 2000, Marstedt and Moebus 2002)? Ernst (2000) found 12 primary studies on the prevalence of CAM with representative surveys among the population. As in the present research, prevalence varied widely between 9% and 65%. He concluded that CAM is used frequently and increasingly, even though its true prevalence remains uncertain as many studies do not sufficiently consider important factors such as the definition of CAM.

A study conducted by the Robert Koch Institute and the German Statistical Office[1] on the use of CAM in Germany also shows that strata with higher education and income levels, as well as women, tend to use CAM more (Marstedt and Moebus 2002). Prevalence also grew strongly from 52% in 1970 to 73% in 2002, which means that three quarters of Germans are using CAM. The intensity of use has also risen; 72% of Germans wish for CAM as a complement to conventional medicine. The survey concludes a very high satisfaction with CAM, even higher than with conventional medicine, although many respondents thought it too dangerous to forgo COM in cases of severe disease. CAM effectiveness was also rated high. The main reasons for using CAM were: dissatisfaction with effectiveness and avoidance of side effects of conventional medicine, self-medication, prevention, closer communication with the therapists.

Both surveys essentially confirm the results of the present research.

7.5   Conclusion

It can be said that CAM therapies play an important part in the countries examined. The question of whether CAM is used as a substitute, addition or complement to COM cannot be answered conclusively on the basis of the study data evaluated. It would be desirable for future studies to investigate this important aspect using a more precise definition and a clearer delineation of concepts.

It can be said in general that the use of CAM methods is very high, with an estimated average 1-year prevalence of one third and lifetime prevalence of two thirds of the respondents. On top of that, the use of CAM has increased over the past years. The majority of respondents find CAM therapies effective.

---

1   Statistisches Bundesamt

7.6   References

Al-Windi A, Elmfeldt D, Svardsudd K (2000) The relationship between age, gender, well-being and symptoms, and the use of pharmaceuticals, herbal medicines and self-care products in a Swedish municipality. Eur J Clin Pharmacol 56:311–317

Anderson DL, Shane-McWhorter L, Crouch BI, Andersen SJ (2000) Prevalence and patterns of alternative medication use in a university hospital outpatient clinic serving rheumatology and geriatric patients. Pharmacotherapy 20:958–966

Armishaw J, Grant CC (1999) Use of complementary treatment by those hospitalized with acute illness. Arch Dis Child 81:133–137

Atteslander P (1993) Methoden der empirischen Sozialforschung. de Gruyter, Berlin/New York

Bortz J (2004) Lehrbuch der empirischen Forschung für Sozialwissenschaftler. Springer-Verlag, Berlin Heidelberg

Brown CM, Segal R (1996) The effects of health and treatment perceptions on the use of prescribed medication and home remedies among African-American and white American hypertensives. Soc Sci Med 43:903–917

Davis MP, Darden PM (2003) Use of complementary and alternative medicine by children in the United States. Arch Pediatr Adolesc Med 157:393–396

Dinehart SM, Alstadt K (2002) Use of alternative therapies by patients undergoing surgery for nonmelanoma skin cancer. Dermatol Surg 28:443–446

Dixon A, Riesberg A, Weinbrenner S, Saka O, Le Grand J, Busse R (2003) Complementary and alternative medicine in the UK and Germany – research and evidence on supply and demand. Anglo-German Foundation for the Study of Industrial Society/Deutsch-Britische Stiftung für das Studium der Industriegesellschaft. London, Berlin. available at: http://www.mig.tu-berlin.de/files/2003.publications/2003.dickson_CAM.report.2003.pdf

Drivdahl CE, Miser W (1998) The use of alternative health care by a family practice population. J Am Board Fam Pract 11:193–199

Eisenberg DM, Davis RB, Ettner SL, Appel S, Wilkey S, Van Rompay M, Kessler RC (1998) Trends in alternative medicine use in the United States, 1990–1997: results of a follow-up national survey. JAMA 280:1569–1575

Eisenberg DM, Kessler RC, Foster C, Norlock FE, Calkins DR, Delbanco TL (1993) Unconventional medicine in the United States: prevalence, costs and patterns of use. N Engl J Med 28:246–252

Elder NC, Gillcrist A, Minz, R (1997) Use of alternative health care by family practice patients. Arch Fam Med 6:181–184

Ernst E, White A (2000) The BBC survey of complementary medicine use in the UK. Complement Ther Med 8:32–36

Ernst E (2000) Prevalence of use of complementary/alternative medicine: a systematic review. Bull World Health Organ 78:252–257

Fairfield KM, Eisenberg DM, Davis RB, Libman H, Phillips RS (1998) Patterns of use, expenditures, and perceived efficacy of complementary and alternative therapies in HIV-infected patients. Arch Intern Med 158: 2257–2264

Foster DF, Phillips RS (2000) Alternative medicine use in older americans. J Am Geriatr Soc 48:1560–1565

Friedrichs J (1980) Methoden empirischer Sozialforschung. Westdeutscher Verlag GmbH, Opladen

Furler MD, Einarson TRW Use of complementary and alternative medicine by HIV-infected outpatients in Ontario, Canada. AIDS Patient Care & STDs 2003 17:155–168

Giese L (2000) A study of alternative health care use for gastrointestinal disorders. Gastroenterol Nursing 23:19–27

Gray CM, Tan AW, Pronk NP, O'Connor PJ (2002) Complementary and alternative medicine use among health plan members. A cross-sectional survey. Effective clinical practice ECP 5:17–22

Haetzman M, Elliott AM, Smith BH, Hannaford P, Chambers WA (2003) Chronic pain and the use of conventional and alternative therapy. Fam Pract 20:147–154

Haltenhof H, Hesse B, Buhler KE (1995) Beurteilung und Verbreitung komplementärmedizinischer Verfahren – eine Befragung von 793 Ärzten in Praxis und Klinik. Gesundheitswesen 57:192–195

Hanyu Ni, Simile C, Hardy AM (2002) Utilization of complementary and alternative medicine by United States adults – results from the 1999 National Health Interview Survey. Med Care 40:353–358

Hayes KM (2000) Alternative therapies and nurse practitioners: knowledge, professional experience, and personal use. Holistic Nursing Pract 14:49–58

Hentschel C, Lindner M, Brinkhaus B, Nagel MR, Hahn EG, Kohnen R (1996) ICD-Diagnosen in einer naturheilkundlichen universitären poliklinischen Sprechstunde. Versicherungsmedizin 48:129–133

Hsiao A-F, Wong M, Kanouse D (2003) Complementary and alternative medicine use and substitution for conventional therapy by HIV-infected patients. J Acquir Immune Defic Syndr 33:157–165

Kaboli P, Doehmer B (2001) Use of complementary and alternative medicine by older patients with arthritis: a population-based study. Arthritis Care Res 45:398–403

Kappauf H, Leykauf-Ammon D, Bruntsch U, Horneber M, Kaiser G, Buschel G, Gallmeier WM (2000) Use of and attitudes held towards unconventional medicine by patients in a department of internal medicine/oncology and haematology. Support Care Cancer 8:314–322

Kemper KJ, Wornham WL (2001) Consultations for holistic pediatric services for inpatients and outpatient oncology patients at a children's hospital. Arch Pediatr Adolesc Med 155:449–454

Kessler RC, Davis RB, Foster DF, Van Rompay MI, Walters EE, Wilkey SA, Kaptchuk TJ, Eisenberg DM (2001) Long-term trends in the use of complementary and alternative medical therapies in the United States. Ann Intern Med 135:262–268

Kessler R, Soukup J (2001) The use of complementary and alternative therapies to treat anxiety and depression in the United States. Am J Psychiatry 158:289–294

Kindermann A (1998) Warum lassen sich Patienten in einer Klinik für TCM behandeln? Hippokrates, Stuttgart

Langmead L, Chitnis M, Rampton DS (2002) Use of complementary therapies by patients with IBD may indicate psychosocial distress. Inflamm Bowel Dis 8:174–179

Lee MM, Chang JS, Jacobs B, Wrensch MR (2002) Complementary and alternative use among men with prostate cancer in 4 ethnic populations. Am J Public Health 92:1606–1609

Marstedt G, Moebus S (2002) Gesundheitsberichterstattung des Bundes Heft 9: Inanspruchnahme alternativer Methoden in der Medizin. Verlag Robert Koch Institut, Berlin

Matthees BJ, Anantachoti P (2001) Use of complementary therapies, adherence, and quality of life in lung transplant recipients. Heart Lung 30:258–268

McFarland B, Bigelow D, Zani B, Newsom J, Kaplan M (2002) Complementary and alternative medicine use in Canada and the United States. Am J Public Health 92:1616–1618

Melchart D, Linde K, Liao JZ, Hager S, Weidenhammer W (1997) Systematic clinical auditing in complementary medicine: rationale, concept, and a pilot study. Altern Ther Health Med 3:33–39

Menniti-Ippolito F, Forcella E, Bologna E, Gargiulo L, Traversa G, Raschetti R (2002) Use of unconventional medicine in children in Italy. Eur J Pediatr 161:690

Messerer M, Johansson SE, Wolk A (2001) Sociodemographic and health behaviour factors among dietary supplement and natural remedy users. Eur J Clin Nutr 55:1104–1110

Messerer M, Johansson SE, Wolk A (2001) Use of dietary supplements and natural remedies increased dramatically during the 1990s. J Intern Med 250:160–166

Norred C (2002) Complementary and alternative medicine use by surgical patients. AORN J 76:1013–1021

Palinkas L, Kabongo M (2000) The use of complementary and alternative medicine by primary care patients: a surf-net study. J Fam Pract 49:1121–1130

Peter S von, Ting W (2002) Survey on the use of complementary and alternative medicine among patients with headache syndromes. Cephalalgia 22:395–400

Pitetti R, Singh S (2001) Complementary and alternative medicine use in children. Pediatr Emerg Care 17:165–169

Premik M (1998) Alternative medicine in Slovenia: some social-medical views. Health Care Anal 6:59–64

Rajendran PR, Thompson RE, Reich SG (2001) The use of alternative therapies by patients with Parkinson's disease. Neurology 57:790–794

Schäfer T, Riehle A, Wichmann HE, Ring J (2002) Alternative medicine in allergies – prevalence, patterns of use, and costs. Allergy 57:694–700

Schnell R, Hill P, Esser E (2004) Methoden der empirischen Sozialforschung. 6th edn. R. Oldenbourg Verlag, Munich Vienna

Sharples FM, van Haselen R, Fisher P (2003) NHS patients' perspective on complementary medicine: a survey. Complement Ther Med 11:243–248

Shenfield G, Lim E, Allen H (2002) Survey of the use of complementary medicines and therapies in children with asthma. J Pediatr Child Health 38:252–257

Unützer J, Klap R, Sturm R, Young AS, Marmon T, Shatkin J, Wells KB (2000) Mental disorders and the use of alternative medicine: results from a national survey. Am J Psychiatry 157:1851–1857

Wang Y, Hashimoto S (1999) A pilot study of the use of alternative medicine in multiple sclerosis patients with special focus on acupuncture. Neurology 52 [Suppl 2]:550

Wellhöfer PR (1997) Grundstudium Sozialwissenschaftliche Methoden und Arbeitsweisen, 2nd edn. Enke Verlag, Stuttgart

Wilkinson JM, Simpson MD (2001) Complementary therapy use by nursing, pharmacy and biomedical science students. Nursing Health Sci 3:19–27

Wilkinson JM, Simpson MD (2001) High use of complementary therapies in a New South Wales rural community. Aust J Rural Health 9:166–171

Wolsko P, Eisenberg D (2003) Patterns and perceptions of care for treatment of back and neck pain: results of a national survey. Spine 28:292–297

Yeh GY, Eisenberg DM (2002) Use of complementary and alternative medicine among persons with diabetes mellitus: results of a national survey. Res Pract 92:1648–1652

Yoon SL, Horne CH (2001) Herbal products and conventional medicines used by community residing older women. J Adv Nursing 33:51–59

7

CAM Conditions and Use in Switzerland

Ursula Wolf, Martin Wolf, Klaus v. Ammon

8.1   Conditions

The generally high acceptance of complementary medicine (VSAO Berne 1988, Jenny et al. 2002) and the particular demand for five complementary medical specialities led to the appointment of a university chair for natural medicine in Zurich in 1994/1995 and, due to a people's initiative, to the installation of a chair with a partial professorship for homeopathy at Bern University (KIKOM)[1].

Almost 140 years following the foundation of the Swiss Association of Homeopathic Physicians (SVHA[2]), one of the oldest physicians' associations in the country, homeopathy was granted minimal academic recognition in Switzerland. Around 400 practising homeopaths are SVHA members, with 296 of them holding the SVHA/FMH[3] homeopathy certificate. The Swiss physicians' society for homeopathy (SAHP[4]) has around 150 members including approximately 100 physicians, 25 of whom are also SVHA members, and around 50 pharmacists. Some practitioners are represented in the Registry of Empirical Medicine (EMR[5]) which assesses mostly non-medical practitioners for registration (quality control) and reimbursement from additional insurance; this will not be considered here.

From 1 July 1999 to 30 June 2005, homeopathic therapies were temporarily included in the statutory Swiss health insurance scheme (KVG[6]) following the decision of the Swiss Federal Council in 1998.

Swiss statutory health insurance is tied to the certificate of competence for homeopathy, which is granted by the SVHA as a diploma and since the beginning of 1999 by the SVHA on behalf of the FMH. Being granted the certificate of competence presupposes a Swiss or recognized foreign specialist physician's qualification. It requires additional homeopathic training ($\geq$400 hours) over a minimum of 4 years and 2 years of homeopathic practice as well as a specialist examination and case documentations, followed by ongoing further training ($\geq$150 hours in 3 years).

The further homeopathic training for physicians is held in accordance with SVHA regulations in all national languages in Zurich, Bern, Lausanne/Geneva and Locarno. Some other further training courses gain part or full recognition in individual cases but are less important.

The practice of homeopathy is based on the classical approach of Hahnemann (from 1796), Bönninghausen (from 1846) and Kent (from 1897) and is extended by more recent practical knowledge. Following registration of the totality of symptoms, single remedies are administered in a strictly individualized fashion, often in high potencies. In the realm of qualified medical homeopathy in Switzerland, complex homeopathy as practiced predominantly in France and Germany and less individualized homeopathic approaches such as clinical homeopathy, 'organotropic' homeopathy and isopathy are of little importance.

The regional distribution of practices in Switzerland shows clear conglomerations around towns and a lack of provision in Southern and Eastern parts of the country (Frei 1999). The concentration of homeopathic provision ranges from 0 in the cantons of Appenzell-Innerrhoden (AI), Jura (JU), Nidwalden (NW) and Uri (UR) to over 40 practising homeopathic physicians per canton (BS – Basel-City, GE – Geneva, ZH – Zurich). It needs to be taken into account that

---

1   KIKOM – Kollegiale Instanz für Komplementärmedizin (Institute for Complementary Medicine)
2   SVHA – Schweizerischer Verein homöopathischer Ärzte und Ärztinnen
3   FMH – Foederatio Medicorum Helveticorum
4   SAHP – Schweizer Ärztegesellschaft für Homöopathie
5   EMR – Erfahrungsmedizinisches Register
6   KVG – Krankenversicherungsgesetz

some cantons, AI (Appenzell Innerrhoden) for instance, have a strong tradition of natural medicine and a corresponding supply of non-medical practitioners. Practice structures, full- and part-time practices, and the percentage of homeopathy used in everyday practice vary strongly.

As far as hospitals are concerned, only the oncology department of the Clinica Santa Croce in Locarno and partly also the Aeskulap Clinic in Brunnen work in the classical homeopathic way at present. The Bircher-Benner Clinic in Zurich and the local hospital in Bauma closed down recently, while the Merian Iselin Hospital in Basle was placed under conventional direction some time ago.

The supply of medicines according to the German Homoeopathic Pharmacopoeia (HAB[7] 2000) is guaranteed either through pharmacies or by direct shipment from specialized Swiss manufacturers, some of which look back on a long manufacturing tradition and a corresponding range of remedies. Sales have to comply with current tariff requirements (*tarif médicale*: TARMED, adopted by the KVG on 1 January 2004). Medicines are listed in the speciality index of the Federal Office of Public Health (FOPH). Some are directly imported from the EU. The systematic adaptation of remedy expiry dates to pharmaceutical standards stands in opposition to homeopathic experience. It is therefore not practice relevant and can, in the view of the speciality associations, put prompt supply in jeopardy. Availability of the whole range of homeopathic remedies has recently also been restricted by the Swiss Agency for Therapeutic Products (Swissmedic), the German Federal Health Office (BGA[8]) and the European Health Office due to the discussion about the biological safety of original substances, especially in the case of nosodes (BSE, sterilisation).

Until 1995, homeopathic research along conventional medical lines was conducted only within the context of bibliographical and editorial studies, some dissertations, publications in specialist journals, and monographs (Righetti 1988, Righetti 1991). Fundamental research and drug research are essential parts of intrinsic homeopathic research. Since the foundation of the KIKOM in Bern, there has been a working group on 'Fundamental research in homeopathy and anthroposophic medicine' (Baumgartner 1998). As a result of an interdisciplinary cooperation a few dissertations (Frei 1999, Wicki 2002) and diploma theses (health care management: Kaiser 1997, Leis 2003) have been completed and some scientific papers have been published in indexed journals (Thurneysen et al. 1994–2004). Other clinical research is rare (Frei and Thurneysen 2001a,b, Hochstrasser and Mattmann 1999). The successful introduction of a consulting service at Bern Inselspital has made the cooperation with clinical and theoretical institutes of the university clinics possible, which again allows for interdisciplinary research work to be carried out that meets all conventional research standards without abandoning essential homeopathic therapy principles (Frei and Thurneysen 2001b, Frei et al. 2004).

Summary

Medical homeopathy is of a high standard in Switzerland and has been provisionally included in the Swiss statutory health insurance scheme (KVG) alongside conventional medical methods. The status is justified by the high demand on the part of the population. The time frame of this temporary provision obligation (6 years) is very tight, given that during that time period an adequate methodology (Heusser 2001) has to be developed and applied to effectively compare systems (evidence of efficacy, appropriateness and economy), although homeopathy does not feature the necessary research structures.

---

7   HAB – Homöopathisches Arzneibuch
8   BGA – Bundesamt für Gesundheit (Germany)

The provision of homeopathic health care is not adequate, especially not in rural areas. Even in towns where the provision is good, demand exceeds supply, which can manifest in long waiting lists.

The supply of remedies is regulated by the Swiss Agency for Therapeutic Products, *swissmedic*, and basically covered by manufacturers in Switzerland. Recently introduced regulations on expiry dates and biological safety are a threat to the homeopathic stock of remedies.

Homeopathy does not have enough academic presence (only a quarter professorship at Bern University), especially as the chair is underequipped for teaching and research and there is no large-scale industrial support. The results from cooperative research are encouraging.

8.2   The Use of Complementary Medicine in Switzerland: Prevalence, Effectiveness, Acceptance and the Views of Patients and Physicians

8.2.1   Introduction

The scientific and statistical evidence arising from the investigation of therapeutic methods that was conducted as part of the complementary medicine programme is supplemented in this chapter by the data retrieved in surveys carried out among the population with regard to experience with and evaluation of complementary and alternative medicine (CAM).

The assessment, on the basis of the literature, of the views of patients and physicians about CAM helps to provide a clearer picture of the needs, wishes and requirements among the population. For this reason interviews were evaluated that explored the prevalence, use, effectiveness and acceptance of CAM, as well as the attitudes of patients and physicians towards it.

8.2.2   Methodology

The literature was searched in the following way: The Index Medicus online (Medline) was searched with the keywords 'complementary medicine, alternative medicine, paramedicine, survey, representative'. The bibliographical reference lists of publications were also searched for further relevant studies. CAM experts and exponents at universities, in hospitals, health insurance companies, patient organisations and pharmaceutical companies were asked for relevant literature. The literature obtained in this way was screened for surveys on the following themes:

- Acceptance of or demand/need for CAM
- Need for a CAM hospital
- Prevalence, use of CAM
- Effectiveness of CAM therapies
- Reimbursement of costs for CAM by health insurers

The literature contained surveys among different populations:

- The general population
- Cancer patients
- Patients with various disorders other than cancer
- Physicians

The data for the four groups were sorted according to the year of the survey. Because CAM is such a comprehensive field, a differentiation between anthroposophically extended medicine, homeopathy, neural therapy, phytotherapy and traditional Chinese medicine was envisaged.

8.2.3 Results

Twenty-four publications were found altogether. The first authors belong to state institutions, universities, medical professional organisations, patient organisations, foundations and health insurance companies. In two cases (Obrist et al. 1990 and Berger et al. 1998, Jenny et al. 2002 and Künzi 2002) surveys were published twice and in one case (Simon 2001, Brander 2001, Wirz 2002) three times and were therefore considered only once in the calculation. Sixteen publications dealt with prevalence, six with acceptance of or the wish for CAM, two with the wish for a CAM hospital, five with the observed effectiveness and one with the wish for its inclusion into the state health-care scheme.

Of the results, 40% originated in representative surveys among the population, 20% in representative surveys among physicians, 30% came from patients in a hospital and 5% from a survey of all obstetric institutions in the German-speaking part of Switzerland.

The first study was published in 1981. Since then the number of publications has risen almost exponentially (cf. ◘ Fig. 8.1).

The results of the various surveys are pictured in ◘ Figs. 8.2–8.4. ◘ Figure 8.2 shows the prevalence, ◘ Fig. 8.3 the acceptance and ◘ Fig. 8.4 the effectiveness of CAM. All results are presented as a function of the survey year.

Two studies describe that a majority of the population (53%, Simon 2001 and 55% Jenny et al. 2002) would prefer a hospital with CAM.

The great majority (85%) of the population wishes for CAM to be reimbursed by the statutory health insurance.

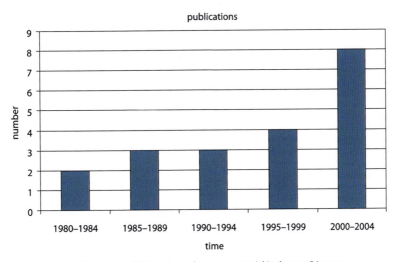

◘ **Fig. 8.1** The increase of surveys on CAM has been almost exponential in the past 24 years

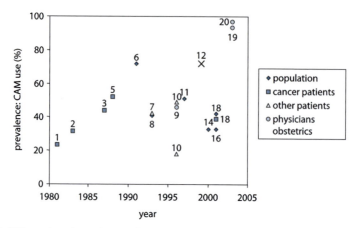

◘ **Fig. 8.2** CAM prevalence/use varies according to the survey theme and population. The values above 80% are from two surveys, one on phytotherapy and one on St. John's wort, both of which are very popular in Switzerland. The value of 18% is the result of a survey in a children's intensive care unit where children and parents received CAM, in 41% of the cases without the knowledge of the physicians in charge. A further 21% of parents would have liked to give CAM but did not do so. The mean value ± standard deviation (SD) of the CAM prevalence is 49 ± 22%. Different symbols were used for the five population subgroups: representative survey among the population (*population*), patients in an oncology clinic (*cancer patients*), patients from other hospitals (*other patients*), representative survey among physicians (*physicians*) and a survey in obstetric institutions (*obstetrics*). Numbers in the diagram refer to the studies (cf. list at the end of this chapter)

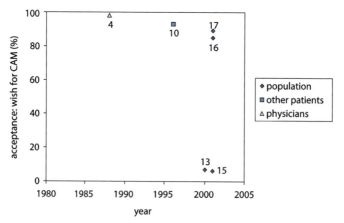

◘ **Fig. 8.3** Over 80% of interviewees expressed acceptance of or the wish for CAM when asked for their opinion on CAM specifically. Values below 10% are from surveys where the population was asked in general about possible improvements in health care without CAM being explicitly mentioned. It is therefore the part of the population that, of their own accord and without being prompted, would see an increased CAM application as an improvement

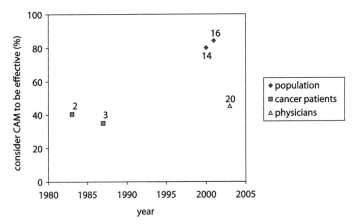

◘ Fig. 8.4 CAM effectiveness judged by cancer patients for their own condition and representative surveys among the population and among physicians regarding the effectiveness of CAM therapies in general. From among the population only actual CAM users were asked. CAM is considered effective by a comparably smaller number of physicians, but it needs to be kept in mind that physicians of all disciplines were asked and not only those who use CAM and have experience with it

8.2.4 Discussion

Each of the questions presented above was part of at least two surveys. The views of the population on CAM are therefore well documented.

In the evaluation and differentiation of the surveys the problem of the CAM definition arose, as it includes a number of different therapies. Some questions referred only to parts of CAM such as phytotherapy or homeopathy. Even when CAM was referred to in general, different approaches were used: Sommer et al. (1996), for instance, listed various kinds of CAM while others asked about CAM use in general.

The survey populations varied between representative surveys and patients with a specific disorder. The duration of use also varied. Questions referred to the previous year or the entire life. All these factors result in a great variability of survey results.

Most publications were found not by screening the Index Medicus Online (Medline) but by searching through bibliographical reference lists and through statements of institutions or individuals in the field of CAM.

8.2.5 Conclusion

About half of the Swiss population have used CAM and value it. About half of the physicians, the great majority of CAM users and ca. 40% of cancer patients consider CAM to be effective. The major part of the population (> 50%) would prefer a CAM hospital. A great majority (85%) of the population would like to have CAM included in the national health insurance scheme.

8.2.6 List of study numbers (referred to in the diagrams)

1. Hauser 1981
2. Obrist et al. 1986
3. Obrist et al. 1990
   Berger et al. 1989 (double publication)
4. VSAO Newsletter 1988
5. Morant et al. 1991
6. Meier and Grau 1992
7. Kranz 1997
8. Sommer et al. 1996
9. Domenighetti et al. 2000
10. Moenkhoff et al. 1999
11. Guillot and Domenighetti 1997
12. Wicki-Frey 2002
13. Brunner et al. 2003
14. Simon 2001
    Brander 2001
    Wirz 2002 (triple publication)
15. Health Office Canton Zurich 2002
16. Jenny et al. 2002
    Künzi 2002 (double publication)
17. Leuenberger et al. 2001
18. van der Weg and Streuli 2003
19. Bachmann and Abt 2003
20. Zeller AG 2003

8.3 References

Bachmann C, Abt C (2003) Das Image der Phytotherapie bei der Schweizer Ärzteschaft: Ergebnisse der Ärzte-Befragung im Mai 2003. Phytotherapie 4:3–4

Baumgartner S, Heusser P, Thurneysen A (1998) Methodological standards and problems in preclinical homeo-pathic potency research. Forschende Komplementärmedizin und klassische Naturheilkunde 5:27–32

Berger DP, Obrist R, Obrecht JP (1989) Tumorpatienten und Paramedizin. Versuch einer Charakterisierung von Anwendern unkonventioneller Therapieverfahren in der Onkologie. Dtsch Med Wochenschr 114:323–330

Brander M (2001) Medienkonferenz Komplementärmedizin im Trend: die Hälfte der Schweizer Bevölkerung wünscht CM Spitäler. Aeskulap-Klinik Klinik press conference, opinion survey of Polyquest. Brunnen

Brunner A, Sabariego TC, Wildner M (2003) Weiterentwicklung des Gesundheitswesens aus Bürgersicht: Ergebnisse einer repräsentativen Bevölkerungsbefragung in München, Dresden, Wien und Bern. Soz Praventiv-med 48:115–120

Domenighetti G, Grilli R, Guillod O, Gutzwiller F, Quaglia J (2000) Usage personnel des pratiques relevant des médecines douces ou alternatives parmi les médecins suisses. Méd Hygiene 58:570–572

Frei H, Everts R, von Ammon K, Kaufmann F, Walter D, Hsu Schmitz SF, Collenberg M, Fuhrer K, Hassink R, Steinlin M, Thurneysen A (2005) Homeopathic treatment of children with attention deficit hyperactivity disorder. Eur J Pediatr 164:758–767

Frei H, Thurneysen A (2001a) Homeopathy in acute otitis media in children: treatment effect or spontaneous resolution? Br Homeopathic J 90:180–182

Frei H, Thurneysen A (2001b) Treatment for hyperactive children: homeopathy and methylphenidate compared in a family setting. Br Homeopathic J 90:183–188

Frei H (2000) Homöopathische Behandlung der Tonsillopharyngitiden bei Kindern. Schweiz Z GanzheitsMed 12:37–40

Frei MK (1999) Psychosomatische Untersuchungen mit dem klinischen Lüscher-Farbtest bei ausgewählten Allergikerinnen. Dissertation, KIKOM Inselspital, University Bern

Gesundheitsdirektion Kt. Zürich (2002) Zufriedenheit der Bevölkerung mit der Gesundheitsversorgung im Kanton Zürich.

Guillot O, Domenighetti G (1997) Etude sur l'effectivité des normes applicables à la relation patient-médecin. Swiss National Research Foundation Project

Gypser KH (ed) (2000) Bönninghausen's Therapeutisches Taschenbuch (1846). Sonntag, Stuttgart

Hahnemann S (1999) Organon der Heilkunst (1842). Schmidt JM (ed). Haug, Stuttgart

Hauser SP (1981) Krebspatient und Paramedizin, Kontakte, Theorien und Behandlungsweisen. Dissertation, University Zurich

Heusser P (2001) Kriterien zur Beurteilung des Nutzens von kmplementärmedizinischen Massnahmen. Forschende Komplementärmedizin und klassische Naturheilkunde 8:14–23

Hochstrasser B, Mattmann P (1999) Mainstream medicine versus complementary medicine (homeopathic) intervention: a critical methodological study of care in pregnancy. Forschende Komplementärmedizin 6 [Suppl 1]: 20–22

Jenny S, Simon M, Meier B (2002) Haltung der Bevölkerung gegenüber der Komplementärmedizin .Schweiz Z GanzheitsMed 14:340–347

Kaiser C (2005) Integration Komplementärmedizin im Regionalspital (Bauma). Diplomarbeit Management im Gesundheitswesen, University Bern

Kent JT (1996) Zur Theorie der Homöopathie (1897). Haug, Stuttgart

Kranz R (1997) Über die Motivation zur Verwendung alternativ-medizinischer Heilmethoden. Dissertation, University Bern

Künzi M (2002) Repräsentative Bevölkerungsbefragung. Die ärztliche Komplementärmedizin ist wirksam! Press release Forschungsstiftung Komplementärmedizin

Leis B, Thurneysen A (2003) Komplementärmedizin. In: Zenger CA, Jung T (eds) Management im Gesundheitswesen und in der Gesundheitspolitik. Hans Huber, Bern, pp 47–56

Leuenberger P, Longchamp C, Bösch L, Golder L, Ratelband-Pally S (2001) Was erwartet die Bevölkerung von der Medizin? gfs Forschungsinstitut www.gfs.ch pp 1–9

Meier V, Grau P (1992) Alternativmedizin – ihre Denkweisen und AnwenderInnen. Perspektiven. Zeichen und Signale/Krankenkasse KKB p 3

Moenkhoff M, Baenziger O, Fischer J, Fanconi S (1999) Parental attitude towards alternative medicine in the paediatric intensive care unit. Eur J Pediatr 158:12–17

Morant R, Jungi WF, Koehli C, Senn HJ (1991) Warum benützen Tumorpatienten Alternativmedizin. Swiss Med Weekly 121:1029–1034

Obrist R, Berger DP, Obrecht JP (1990) Attitude of ambulatory oncological patients to academic medicine, their physician and nurse. Results of an anonymous survey. Schweiz RundschMed Prax 79:416–419

Obrist R, von Meiss M, Obrecht JP (1986) Verwendung paramedizinischer Behandlungsmethoden durch Tumorpatienten. Dtsch Med Wochenschr 111:283–287

Righetti M (1991) Characteristics and selected results of research in homeopathy. Berlin J Res Homeopathy 1:195–203

Righetti M (1988) Forschung in der Homöopathie. Burgdorf, Göttingen

Sankaran R (1991) The spirit of homeopathy. Homeopathic Medical Publishers, Bombay

Simon M (2001)Medienkonferenz Komplementärmedizin im Trend: Einstellung der Bevölkerung gegenüber der Komplementärmedizin. Aeskulap-Klinik press conference, opinion survey of Polyquest. Brunnen

Sommer JH, Bürgi M, Theiss R (1996) Verbreitung alternativer Heilmethoden in der Schweiz – Eine empirische Untersuchung. Forschende Komplementärmedizin 3:289–299

Thurneysen et al. (2004) persönliche Mitteilung, KIKOM, Bern

van der Weg F, Streuli RA (2003) Use of alternative medicine by patients with cancer in a rural area of Switzerland. Swiss Med Weekly 133:233–240

Verband Schweizerischer Assistenz- und Oberärztinnen und -ärzte (VSAO) (1988) Auswertung der Umfrage „Alternativmedizin" des VSAO, Sektion Bern. VSAO Newslett 4:10–18

Wicki-Frey G Homöopathie in der Geburtshilfe der Schweiz? Dissertation, Universität Bern, 2002

Wirz U (2002) Her mit der Komplementärmedizin. Prim Care 2:371–374

Zeller AG (2003) Angaben zum Konsum von Phytotherapie in der Schweiz. Zeller Pharma

Overview of Systematic Reviews on the Clinical Efficacy of Homeopathy

Gudrun Bornhöft, Klaus v. Ammon

9.1   Introduction: Systematic Reviews

Systematic reviews are used to filter conclusive, reproducible information – usually concerning the effectiveness of medical interventions – from the overwhelming quantity of individual study results. For this purpose research results are systematically collected, evaluated and summarized. They differ from traditional reviews and expert commentaries in that they have a scientific, transparent and reproducible approach which tries to minimize the risk of bias. Systematic reviews are not so much about reflecting expert opinions; rather, they seek to establish a balanced and neutral reproduction and analysis of the evidence available.

Systematic reviews support the planning of further research, as they not only assess the evidence, but also reveal research flaws. ▪ Table 9.1 explains the different kinds of reviews and overviews:

9.2   Literature Search

Two strategies were used to identify the systematic reviews and meta-analyses available. For homeopathy we used four well-researched reviews of systematic reviews (Linde et al. 2001, Ernst 2002, Jonas et al. 2003 and O'Meara et al. 2003). As the older overview by Linde et al. (2001) is, with 18 reviews, the most comprehensive, we used it to identify reviews published before 2000. Then we screened our own homeopathy literature database, which had been established using the search results of various publically accessible databases (see Chap. 6), with the search terms 'systematic review' and 'meta-analysis' in order to find reviews published after 2000. A total of 356 articles were found. Of these we chose 23 whose titles and/or abstracts seemed relevant to our question. A search through the bibliographical reference lists produced a further 19. Of the

▪ **Table 9.1** Research and review terminology (based on Glanville and Sowden 2001)

Name	Explanation
review	An article that summarizes a number of different primary studies and may draw conclusions about the effectiveness of a particular intervention. A review may or may not be systematic.
systematic review/ systematic overview	A review of the evidence on a clearly formulated question that uses systematic and explicit methods to identify, select and critically appraise relevant primary research, and to extract and analyse data from the studies that are included in the review. Statistical methods (meta-analysis) may or may not be used.
meta-analysis	The use of statistical techniques to combine the results of studies addressing the same question into a summary measure.
health technology assessment (HTA)	Health technology includes any method used by those working in health services to promote health, screen, diagnose, prevent and treat disease, and to improve rehabilitation and long-term care. HTA considers the effectiveness, appropriateness, costs and broader impact of health technologies using both primary research and systematic reviews. It seeks to meet the information needs of those who use these technologies, as well as of those who manage and provide health and social care.

now 60 available articles, 38 were excluded after perusal of their full texts, most of them because they turned out not to be systematic reviews after all. Three of them had also been included in Linde's original review.

The following inclusion and exclusion criteria applied in addition to the general ones set out in Chap. 6:

Inclusion criteria:
- Study design: systematic review or meta-analysis with the provisos: systematic search in adequate databases (at least Medline) with statement of inclusion and exclusion criteria or explicit statement that a systematic search had taken place.
- Publication: the study has been published.

Exclusion criteria:
- Inclusion criteria not met, e.g. no systematic review or review on drug tests
- Research questions not relevant to the present HTA
- Re-analyses, i.e. articles that re-evaluate the data of other reviews. (When the corresponding original reviews were presented, these re-analyses were included as comments.)
- Double publications

See the end of the chapter for a list of excluded studies and the reasons for their exclusion.

9.3 Presentation of the Studies

The 22 review articles which we used are briefly presented here:

9.3.1 Reviews on general effectiveness

1. **Boissel 1996**
   Critical literature review on the effectiveness of homeopathy: Overview of data from homeopathic medicine trials
   Based on the inclusion criteria: controlled studies on human beings, homeopathy and placebo control, 184 clinical studies were subjected to a meta-analysis. Evaluation of all 184 studies showed high significance in favour of homeopathy; for the 17 studies with the highest methodological quality the result was still $p < 0.001$ and only turned to not significant in the sensitivity analysis after another four studies had been excluded.

2. **Cucherat et al. 2000**
   Evidence of clinical efficacy of homeopathy: a meta-analysis of clinical trials
   Seventeen clinical studies (in 16 articles) with a total of 2617 patients were subjected to a meta-analysis with the inclusion criteria: RCT, placebo control and end points as clinical or surrogate parameters. All studies had a combined effect value of $p = 0.000036$ (which indicates the probability of at least one result not being accidentally positive). After restriction to double-blind studies: $p = 0.000068$, after further restriction to studies with loss to follow-up <10%: $p = 0.0084$. Only after restriction to studies with loss to follow-up <5%, p became not significant at 0.082.

3. **Ernst 1999b**
   Classical homeopathy versus conventional treatments: a systematic review
   Six clinical studies were subjected to descriptive analysis, the inclusion criteria being: classical, individualized homeopathy and allopathic control treatment. Four studies showed equivalence or even superiority of the homeopathic compared with the allopathic treatment; two studies were inferior.

4. **Grabia and Ernst 2003**
   Homeopathic aggravations: a systematic review of randomized placebo-controlled clinical trials
   Twenty-five clinical studies involving 3437 patients in total were subjected to descriptive analysis with the inclusion criteria: RCT, double-blind, placebo controlled and therapeutic intervention. There were clearly more indications of aggravations and also adverse effects in the verum group than in the control groups. The result suggests an effectiveness of homeopathic medicines that differs from placebo (cf. Chap. 11).

5. **Hill and Doydon 1990**
   Review of randomized trials of homeopathy
   Forty clinical studies with an average of 28 patients each (median, range: 10–600) were subjected to descriptive analysis with the inclusion criteria: RCT or double-blind. Twenty-one studies showed a positive result in favour of homeopathy, 19 did not; of the three studies with best methodology one was positive, two were not.

6. **Kleijnen et al. 1991**
   Clinical trials of homeopathy
   A total of 107 clinical studies were subjected to descriptive analysis with their own quality assessment, the inclusion criteria being: controlled study on human beings. Fourteen studies were on classical homeopathy, 58 on clinical homeopathy, 26 on complex homeopathy and nine on isopathy; 81 studies showed a positive result in favour of homeopathy, 24 did not (compared with placebo). Of the highest-quality studies (score ≥55) 15 showed significant effects in favour of homeopathy, seven did not.
   Comment:
   This 'milestone' study has had a marked influence on homeopathy research in subsequent years, especially on its literature analyses.
   Because Kleijnen et al. collected such extensive data over a period of 3 years, Ernst and Resch (1996) re-analysed the data to find out whether a simple Medline search would have produced similar results and might therefore have been sufficient. They split the articles of the Kleijnen analysis into two groups, Medline indexed yes or no, and worked out the percentage of positive and negative results. The results were similar, which led the authors to conclude that a Medline search would, in principle, suffice. The 'English language only' restriction is said to lead to publication bias. The authors also found that the results for treatment of chronic disease were more often in favour of homeopathy than those for treatment of acute disease.

7. **Linde et al. 1997**
   Are the clinical effects of homeopathy placebo effects? A meta-analysis of placebo-controlled trials
   Eighty-nine clinical studies were subjected to meta-analysis, the inclusion criteria being: controlled studies on therapy and prevention, placebo controlled, randomized or double-blind and sufficient data for meta-analysis. The combined odds ratio for all 89 studies was OR 2.45 (2.05–2.93, 95% CI) in favour of homeopathy. For the 26 best studies: OR 1.66

(1.33–2.08, 95% CI), after correction of publication bias 1.78 (1.03–3.10, 95% CI). The authors concluded: 'The results do not confirm the null hypothesis that there is no difference between homeopathy and placebo.'

Comment:

The study provoked lively discussion in the journal where it was originally published, *The Lancet*, as well as among the wider public. Apart from the charge of comparing 'apples and pears' due to the very heterogeneous data material, it was also pointed out that the quality of the studies showed an obvious negative correlation to the result, which means that, when interpreting the data, it had to be taken into account that studies of higher quality tended to arrive at a negative result. Linde et al. (1999) decided to re-analyse their own data, applying different quality parameters in univariate and multivariate regression models, and found in fact a tendency for this negative correlation, but no linear relationship; they pointed out that several items and quality values did not support linearity. What is astonishing is the 'decline' in the discussion that followed, where Ernst and Pittler (2000) entered the data into a different scale and postulated a 'negative linearity'. They interpreted the high score of 5 for study quality (Jadad) (which did not fit the picture but was reached by ten of the studies and showed a positive trend for homeopathy) as a 'seemingly convincing, but not creditable'(!) result and declared their re-analysis to be the 'ultimate epidemiological evidence that homeopathic medicines are in fact placebos.' When Lüdtke (2002) pointed out methodological flaws, Ernst admitted to this straight out in his response, which was printed on the same page, claiming that his intention had been to provoke the 'homeopathic camp', but that he still saw a negative linearity after correction of the methodological flaws.

A re-analysis of the Linde study by Ernst (1998) must also be mentioned. Of the literature Linde collected, he subjected only the studies with high potencies, and of these only those with the highest-quality score (≥90 of 100, which is an unusually strict inclusion criterion) to a meta-analysis. The combined *p*-value of the five extremely heterogeneous studies showed no difference to placebo.

8. **Linde and Melchart 1998**
   Randomized Controlled Trials of individualized Homeopathy: A State-of-the-Art Review
   With the inclusion criteria: individualized homeopathy for therapy and prevention and randomized, quasi-randomized or double-blind, 32 clinical studies with altogether 1778 patients (median 44) were subjected to descriptive analysis, 19 of them also to a meta-analysis. The pooled rate ratio was 1.62 (95% CI, 1.17–2.23) and, after restriction to the six studies with the highest methodological quality 1.12 (95% CI, 0.87–1.44). For the category 'unlikely to have major flaws' (another six studies) the result was again significant at 2.44 (95% CI, 1.30–4.59).

9. **Lutz 1993**
   Quantitative Meta-Analyse empirischer Ergebnisse der Homöopathieforschung
   Twenty-two clinical studies with a total of 3105 patients and the inclusion criteria: controlled clinical study on human beings, purely homeopathic remedies and accessibility of the studies, were subjected to descriptive analysis, 14 of them also to a meta-analysis. Four showed a high effect value (≥0.8). With the studies being very inhomogeneous, a combination of effect sizes would not have made sense. There was no correlation between methodological quality and outcome, but there was a negative trend between the 'purity of the homeopathic intervention' (model validity) and effect size.

10. **Walach 1997**

Unspezifische Therapie-Effekte – Das Beispiel Homöopathie

Using as inclusion criteria: RCT, placebo and standard control, adequate statistical evaluation, publication with peer review in non-homeopathic journals accessible via Medline and Embase, 41 clinical studies involving a total of 6163 patients were subjected to descriptive analysis, 23 of them also to a meta-analysis. There was, on the whole, no clear difference between the homeopathic remedy and the placebo, but paradoxically not between homeopathic and standard therapy either. The combined effect size was slightly positive at G=0.29. Variance was very strong, so that an overall population effect size cannot be assumed.

9.3.2 Reviews on special indications:

1. **Barnes et al. 1997**

   Homeopathy for postoperative ileus?

   Six clinical studies involving a total of 776 patients were subjected to descriptive analysis and a meta-analysis, the inclusion criteria being: controlled clinical studies (+ indication: postoperative ileus). Five of the six studies showed a positive result in favour of the homeopathic treatment. The weighted mean difference (WMD) of all six studies with regard to reduced duration of ileus was –7.4 h in favour of homeopathy (95% CI, –4.0 to –10.8 h) with significance $p < 0.05$. The exclusion of low-quality studies made no essential difference in the result. The effect is clinically relevant. Subgroup analysis of low and medium potencies (<C12; four studies) showed a statistically significant WMD of –6.6 h, analysis of high potencies a non-significant trend with a WMD of –3.1 h (95% CI, 1.3 to –7.5 h).

2. **Ernst 1999a**

   Homeopathic prophylaxis of headaches and migraines? A systematic review

   Four clinical studies were subjected to descriptive analysis, the inclusion criteria being: RCT, placebo control and double-blind. One study showed a significant effect in favour of homeopathy in all end points, another one for one of four end points, the other two no or no significant (no differentiation made by author) difference between placebo and verum groups.

3. **Ernst and Barnes 1998**

   Are homeopathic remedies effective for delayed-onset muscle soreness?

   Eight clinical studies were subjected to descriptive analysis, the inclusion criteria being: controlled clinical studies, placebo control, volunteers, double-blind and quantitative end points. The randomized studies showed no difference between verum and placebo groups, while the non-randomized studies (with small numbers of participants) showed significant effects in favour of homeopathy.

   Comment:

   Dean (1998) re-analysed and criticized the Ernst study because (a) not all available studies had been considered, (b) excluding some studies due to insufficient participant numbers seemed unjustified, (c) it had not been fully considered in the discussion and interpretation of results that the significance threshold of $p < 0.05$ was a convention and that it was therefore not right to declare studies with $p = 0.04$ to be positive and those with $p = 0.06$ to be negative, (d) the strong heterogeneity in setting and outcome parameters had not been taken into account (muscle tension always had a positive outcome), and (e) the study design was not compatible with homeopathic practice: although low potencies were suitable for lowest common denominator symptoms, treatment became increasingly specific with increasing potency grades and therefore required more individualisation. Without that, there was a greater risk of missing the therapeutic goal. Fisher (1999) agrees with this re-analysis, but points out that other high-quality studies had not been able to demonstrate effectiveness for Arnica (which might be disappointing for the homeopathic community, but a relief for sports events organizers who otherwise would have been guilty of using an undetectable doping drug – D30).

4. **Jonas et al. 2000**
   Homeopathy and Rheumatic Disease
   A meta-analysis was performed on six clinical studies with a total of 392 patients, the inclusion criteria being: controlled study on therapy and prevention, placebo controlled, randomized or double-blind and sufficient data for a meta-analysis (+ indication). The overall odds ratio (OR) was 2.19 (95% CI, 1.5–.11), for the five methodologically best studies (of six studies in total) OR = 2.11 (95% CI, 1.32–3.35) with a significance of $p = 0.002$. For the two studies with classical individualized therapy ($n = 90$ patients) an OR = 2.04 could be established, but the confidence interval (CI) was very high with values between 0.66 and 6.34 and was below 1, which meant that no reliable effects could be concluded for classical homeopathy.

5. **Linde and Jobst 1998**
   Homeopathy for chronic asthma
   Three clinical analyses were subjected to descriptive analysis, the inclusion criteria being: RCT, homeopathic treatment and asthma. Two of the three studies showed a significantly positive effect in favour of homeopathy; among them was also the study with the highest quality score (even though the effect it showed was of little clinical relevance). The third study showed no difference between the groups.

6. **Long 2001**
   Homeopathic remedies for the treatment of osteoarthritis: a systematic review
   Four clinical studies were subjected to descriptive analysis, the inclusion criteria being: RCT (+ indication). Three studies compared homeopathic remedies with conventional therapies and one with placebo. The latter showed no significant effect, while the comparison with conventional treatment showed equality in two studies and in one study even a trend in favour of homeopathy.

7. **Smith 2001**
   Homeopathy for induction of labour
   A descriptive analysis was carried out of one clinical study involving 40 patients, the inclusion criteria being: RCT, no treatment, placebo or other controls (from a list set out beforehand by the author) and end points according to a panel predefined by the author. Only one study was found that showed no difference between homeopathic treatment (Caulophyllum) and placebo group for the end points cervical ripening and induction of labour.

9.3.3 Reviews on special interventions

1. **Bauer et al. 2002**
   The use of Arnica for the treatment of soft-tissue damage
   Nine clinical studies were subjected to descriptive analysis; three showed results in favour of homeopathy, six did not.

2. **Ernst and Pittler 1998a**
   Efficacy of homeopathic Arnica
   Eight clinical studies were subjected to descriptive analysis, the inclusion criteria being: homeopathy and Arnica. Three showed no difference between verum and placebo, among them also two of the three higher quality studies; five showed a trend in favour of homeopathy.
3. **Lüdtke 1999**
   Klinische Wirksamkeit zu Arnica in homöopathischen Zubereitungen
   Thirty-seven clinical studies were subjected to descriptive and, if sufficient data were available, also to comparative quantitative analysis. Inclusion criteria were: controlled clinical studies, placebo control or no treatment, Arnica montana as single remedy, in combination or as a complex. Thirty-five percent of the studies showed significant superiority for Arnica, including all complex remedies. One study showed significance for the control. A clear correlation between (high) study quality and (negative) outcome could not be established, at most a trend. Over time (i.e. in later publication years) the studies tended to show more significance in favour of homeopathy. The best effect was registered for wound healing, the weakest for muscle soreness.

9.3.3   Reviews on special indications with special intervention

1. **Vickers and Smith 2000**
   Homeopathic Oscillococcinum for preventing and treating influenza and influenza-like syndromes
   Seven clinical studies were subjected to descriptive analysis and a meta-analysis, the inclusion criteria being: placebo control, prophylaxis or therapy with Oscillococcinum, homeopathically prepared influenza viruses, influenza vaccines or chicken liver and influenza or influenza-like syndrome. Three of the studies were on prophylaxis and involved a total of 2265 participants and four were treatment studies involving altogether 1194 participants. The prophylaxis studies showed no superiority of the homeopathic treatment with a relative risk of RR=0.64 (95% CI, 0.28–1.43). In the treatment studies, Oscillococcinum reduced the duration of the illness by 0.28 days (95% CI, 0.5–0.06). The patients' evaluation of effectiveness was in favour of homeopathy with RR=1.08 (95% CI, 1.17–1). In summary, there is no evidence that the homeopathic treatment has a prophylactic effect, but treatment reduces the duration of disease and is seen as more effective by patients.
2. **Wiesenauer and Lüdtke 1996**
   A meta-analysis of the homeopathic treatment of pollinosis with Galphimia glauca
   Eleven clinical studies with a total of 1038 patients were subjected to descriptive analysis and a meta-analysis, the inclusion criteria being: pollinosis, Galphimia glauca and homeopathy. All studies were conducted by the same team of researchers, but at different centres and practices. The success rate of Galphimia was 1.25 times higher than that of placebo (CI 1.09–1.43). The estimated success rate in the verum group was 79.3% (CI: 74.1–85.0 %). The homeopathic treatment with Galphimia was therefore significantly superior to placebo for eye symptoms and apparently equivalent to antihistamine treatment.

9.4 Evaluation of the Studies

The studies were described and evaluated in adherence to the following criteria (adapted from Glanville and Sowden 2001):

- What is the review's **objective**?
- What **sources** were searched to identify primary studies? (What databases and other sources, what search strategies; were any restrictions used as to language, type of study etc.)
- What were the **inclusion and exclusion criteria** and how were they applied?
- What criteria were used to assess the quality of primary studies and how were they applied (e.g. quality score according to Jadad or other **quality criteria**)?
- What **data/information** were/was extracted from the primary studies and how?
- How were the **data synthesized**? (How were differences between studies presented and interpreted? How were the results combined? Was it reasonable to combine them? What are the results of the review? Do the conclusions follow logically from the evidence established?)

The evaluation, i.e. the determination of a study's quality or validity, mostly serves to estimate to what extent the study results and statements are 'correct' or possibly biased due to factors that were not explicitly considered.

As shown in Chap. 5, in addition to the usual internal validity we evaluated the external validity, i.e. whether the study reflects actual practice or whether the study results are transferable to our research question. The two evaluations are therefore listed separately.

9.4.1 Research question

The research questions were presented in Sect. 9.3. An evaluation of the internal validity of the research question was not necessary. As the studies already existed, operationalisability was assumed. The external validity was assessed in three categories: question relevant +, partly

▢ Table 9.2 Summary of the research topics of included reviews with number of primary studies analysed and evaluation of external validity

Question	No. of reviews	No. of studies analysed in the reviews	Ratio of relevant/ restrictedly relevant questions
general effectiveness (all indications, all homeopathic remedies)	10	563	8/2
specific indication	7	32	6/1
specific intervention (homeopathic remedy)	3	54	0/3
specific indication with specific homeopathic remedy	2	18	0/2
Total	22	667	14/8

relevant (+) or not relevant, with the latter serving as an exclusion criterion when the title lists and abstracts were screened.

◼ Table 9.3 lists the studies that were included, with their research subject and an estimation of its relevance.

◼ Table 9.3 Overview of included studies with their research subject, number of analysed studies and evaluation of the external validity (relevance) of the question

Authors, year	No. of studies analysed	No. of patients analysed	Research subject		Evaluation: question relevant '+' or partly relevant '(+)'
			Indication	Intervention	
Barnes et al. 1997	6	776	postoperative ileus	all	+
Bauer et al. 2002	9	n.s.*	all	Arnica	(+)[1]
Boissel 1996	184	n.s.	all	all	+
Cucherat et al. 2000	17	2617	all	all	+
Ernst 1999 a	4	n.s.	headache/ migraine	all	+
Ernst 1999 b	6	n.s.	all	all vs. conventional treatment	+
Ernst and Barnes 1998	8	n.s.	muscle soreness	all, mostly Arnica	(+)[2]
Ernst 1998	8	n.s.	all	Arnica	(+)[1]
Grabia and Ernst 2003	25	3437	all	all	+
Hill and Doyon 1990	40	> 1000	all	all	(+)[3]
Jonas et al. 2000	6	392	rheumatic disease	all	+
Kleijnen et al. 1991	107	n.s.	all	all	+
Linde et al. 1997	89	n.s.	all	all	+
Linde and Jobst 1998	3	n.s.	chronic asthma	all	+
Linde and Melchart 1998	32	1778	all	individualized homeopathy	(+)[3]
Long 2001	4	n.s.	osteoarthritis	all	+
Lüdtke 1999 ▾	37	n.s.	all	Arnica	(+)[1]

◻ **Table 9.3** (continued)

Authors, year	No. of studies analysed	No. of patients analysed	Research subject		Evaluation: question relevant '+' or partly relevant '(+)'
			Indication	Intervention	
Smith 2001	1	40	labour induction	all (Caulophyllum)	+
Vickers 2000	7	3459	influenza	Oscillococcinum	(+)[1]
Walach 1997	41	6163	all	all	+
Wiesenauer and Lüdtke 1996	11	1038	pollinosis (hay fever)	Galphimia glauca	(+)[1]

* n.s: not specified
Reasons for restricted relevance (see also text below):
[1] restriction to one medicine, not individualized
[2] experimental condition (muscle soreness), not relevant to medical practice
[3] restriction to RCTs (see Chap. 5) even with individualized intervention.

Both tables show that almost half of the reviews focus on the general evaluation of homeopathic treatment, which, on the one hand, conforms to the question of the present HTA and is therefore highly relevant for our research and makes it possible, on the other hand, to accommodate the individual variability in matching illness/patient characteristics to a particular homeopathic remedy. This matching of remedy and patient which is part of homeopathic practice is also possible with subgroups, e.g. for special syndromes or symptom complexes. Restriction of the practice relevance, i.e. of the external validity, is therefore greatest for the intervention studies, which were conducted in the attempt to increase the homogeneity of the included studies and thus their comparability (internal validity). This restriction is particularly high for fixed matchings to one indication, because examining the effectiveness of a particular homeopathic medicine without considering the individual compatibility is not in accordance with fundamental homeopathic thinking and acting.

For greater clarity the number of included studies is listed, too. As expected, many more studies were found for the more widely defined research questions (up to 184 in one review) than for restricted topics.

9.4.2 Selection of studies

1. Data sources

Of the 22 reviews 21 included data sources, but only one study named the selection criteria.

The study by Linde et al. (1997) was frequently used as a basis, partly also the older and very comprehensive compilation by Kleijnen et al. (1991). Two studies used only the Linde material and four studies did not mention the databases they searched. Of the remaining 16 studies about two thirds stated that they had screened bibliographical references, half by handsearching CAM journals and one quarter via contacts to manufacturers.

The databases mentioned were, with one exception, retrieved mainly from Medline followed by searches in the following databases (partial overlapping accounts for sum total ≥16):

	Times mentioned
Medline	15
Embase	11
Cochrane Library	9
Amed	5
Ciscom	5
Cinahl	4
British Library Stock Alert	4
PsychInfo	3
Biosis	3
Complem. Med. Index	3
Science Citation Index	2
HomInfo	2
Register Woodward Foundation	1
IDAG	1
Econlit	1
ZETOC	1

Search strategies were specified in about half, the time period assessed in ca. two thirds of the studies.

We assessed the finding of data/data sources together with the general evaluation of the study design in terms of reproducibility and sufficient documentation (internal validity). Interpretation with regard to the external validity (contact with experts, hand search, search in CAM-oriented databases such as Amed) was considered to be speculative and therefore omitted, especially as there was no information on how many studies were in fact accessed via which sources. (A paper by Ernst 1996 suggests that the qualitative outcome is biased only minimally through restriction to the most common database, Medline.)

2. Inclusion and exclusion criteria

In ten of the 22 studies inclusion criteria were fully documented, in two of them partly. Only one review where a systematic search was explicitly mentioned supplied no inclusion and exclusion criteria.

The selection criteria often constituted the key research points as in the case of a special indication or intervention.

When evaluating internal and external validity with regard to the selection of studies, a discrepancy between these two validity categories is possible. While internal validity needs the highest possible homogeneity in the comparison groups (in terms of composition and treatment) which is best achieved with restrictive inclusion and exclusion criteria, randomisation and blinding, this does not do justice to the real practice situation – a fact which, in principle, applies to any medical treatment, be it conventional or complementary. Especially with a complementary medical method such as homeopathy one has to assume, however, that patients consciously decide in favour of it, which means the study results do not transfer easily from RCTs to the real-life situation in homeopathy, which is being investigated here, and the results

⬛ Table 9.4 Overview of study types as inclusion criterion

Inclusion criterion	Number of reviews
RCT or double blind	10
controlled clinical studies without explicit randomisation criterion	8
no explicit restriction to particular study types	1

can hardly reflect the actual conditions of homeopathy usage. The relevant inclusion criteria (named in 19 studies) are set out in ⬛ Table 9.4.

Of the eight reviews that included only controlled studies without explicitly specifying randomisation as a criterion, four listed as an inclusion criterion placebo control, which usually comes with randomisation and blinding. One review selected only studies with a conventional control, while three left the kind of control open.

Two (of 22) studies mentioned individualized classical homeopathic therapy as a further practice-relevant inclusion criterion.

To summarize: there were only three reviews with high external validity of study selection due to explicit inclusion criteria (individualisation) or due to their openness regarding the study types they included. Ten other studies probably traded in their high internal validity (greatest possible comparability of groups through randomisation) for external validity.

From the homeopathic point of view, conventional quality criteria cannot necessarily be transferred to homeopathic studies without adaptation:

— In most cases, placebo-controlled, blinded homeopathy studies limit the external validity. Conventional medicine examines the specific effect of a pharmaceutical substance, while the homeopathic substance does not have an effect per se; rather the effect arises from its complex individual interaction with the organism. Before the substance that is indicated in the individual case can be gleaned from the Materia Medica, a complex process of history-taking, observation and self-observation of the individual symptoms has to take place. How long a medicinal effect lasts is also individually different. With the exception of very simple cases, the treatment controls become too confusing if it is uncertain whether the patient has received a placebo or a wrong/not optimal remedy and whether that remedy is still having an effect or not.

— Further factors would need to be observed and described in correct studies, e.g. full individualisation or preselection of medication, antidoting, inclusion and exclusion criteria from the homeopathic point of view (e.g. reaction block due to certain medicaments, drugs, severe organ disease, condition after surgery), individual remedy repetition depending on reaction and effect duration, adequate length of observation period (especially for chronic disease).

9.4.3 Selection and evaluation of data/information

The kind of information extracted from the studies strongly depends on the chosen quality criteria. The reviews investigated again focused almost exclusively on internal validity, which means that – next to information on the study character (PICO: population, intervention, control, outcome parameters as well as the results in themselves) – mostly data on randomisation, blinding and loss rate (dropout, loss to follow-up) were extracted to assess the known bias factors (selection, performance, attrition and detection) (see Chap. 5.2).

Data that would be relevant for the evaluation of external validity such as the following are not usually documented.

- Intervention: assessment of parameters relevant for the evaluation of external validity (e.g. individualized therapy for homeopathy)?
- Population: assessment of parameters besides indication (e.g. patient recruitment etc.)?
- Performance: assessment of the qualification of treating physicians?
- End points: is there an obvious differentiation of clinical parameters, surrogate parameters and quality of life?
- Results: consideration of the clinical relevance of effects?
- Safety: assessment and adequate homeopathic evaluation of 'adverse events' – initial aggravation; symptom progression according to Hering's rule?
- Follow-up: assessment of follow-up time with adequate evaluation in relation to the disease?

If they were mentioned in exceptional cases, they were usually not included in the actual quality assessment.

Fifteen of the 22 studies named criteria for their quality assessment, 13 of them only internally valid ones. Six of those applied the Jadad Score, either by itself or in combination with other criteria of internal validity.

Only two included externally valid criteria as well, but they hardly figured in the subsequent data synthesis (see ◘ Fig. 9.1).

9.4.4 Data synthesis

Glanville and Sowden (2001) consider the following questions to be central in the evaluation of the data synthesis:

1. How are the differences in individual study results presented and interpreted?
2. How are the study results synthesized?
3. What are the study results?
4. Do the final conclusions follow from the evidence?

Ad 1: differences in study results: there are different ways of dealing with different study results. The simplest way (which also has severe error potential) is to contrast the number of positive

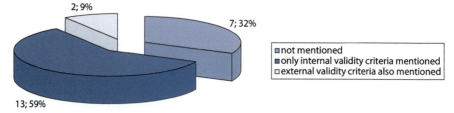

◘ Fig 9.1 Information on quality criteria used in the reviews investigated: seven did not mention any, 13 mentioned only internal validity criteria, two mentioned additional external validity criteria

Table 9.5 Distribution of methods used for data synthesis	
Data synthesis methods	No. of reviews
only quantitative (meta-analysis)	3
quantitative and qualitative	7
only qualitative (descriptive)	11
simple vote count (exclusively)	1

and negative studies without comment as vote counts and use the arithmetic mean as the result. A less formalized, but obviously more appropriate way is to separate the differences according to content and base the overall conclusion on preferably pre-defined criteria. This can be done in more or less formalized ways. It is common to use quality criteria to create subgroups and to 'seriously' consider only the studies with the highest-quality score as their results were presumably least affected by bias.

Ad 2:. Analysis and synthesis of results can happen in a descriptive, qualitative or quantitative form through meta-analysis. The latter has the advantage that it is able to statistically evaluate data from several smaller studies in a combined result. What speaks against it is that it compares 'apples and pears' – due to the heterogeneity of data which cannot be avoided even by heterogeneity testing and selection of suitable analysis models – and that it suggests a pseudo-accuracy which does not actually correspond to the data. ◻ Table 9.5 lists the distribution of the methods used for data synthesis:

Ad 3 and 4: Results and conclusion. The quantitative and qualitative results are given in the presentation of reviews at the beginning of this chapter.
　　◻ Table 9.6 offers a schematic view of study results with the conclusions and rationale of the authors and our own evaluations (with reasons for difference, if applicable).
　　An obvious discrepancy between the study results as such and their frequent downgrading by the authors was noticeable in 15 reviews. Wherever the downgrading was explained with very strict internal validity criteria we usually overruled it, as it is the aim of the present HTA to evaluate effectiveness in the reality of health-care provision (where patients consciously – without randomisation – decide in favour of homeopathic treatment and know – without blinding – which remedies they are given), which means that the strong emphasis on randomisation and blinding holds too high a risk of false-negative results (cf. Chaps. 5 and 13). We overruled the downgrading in ten cases but also graded two studies lower than the authors had done.

■ Table 9.6 Summary of study results, authors' conclusions and our own evaluation

Author, year	Result	Conclu-sion	Authors' rationale	Own conclusion	Reasons
Barnes et al. 1997	+	(+)	reservations not explained	+	reservations not shared
Bauer et al. 2002	∅	∅	n.c.	(+)	pos. and neg. results don't balance each other out
Boissel 1996	+/(+)	(+)	low quality	(+)	n.c.
Cucherat et al. 2000	+/(+)	(+)	low quality	+	dropout <5% too strict, significance up to 10%
Ernst 1999 a	+/(+)	∅	vote count	(+)	pos. and neg. results don't balance each other out
Ernst 1999 b	+	∅	methodologi-cal flaws	(+)	reservations not shared; few data
Ernst and Barnes 1998	∅/(+)	∅	methodologi-cal flaws	∅	n.c.
Ernst 1998	(+)/∅	∅	no effect in more rigorous studies	(+)	very restrictive rationale not shared
Grabia and Ernst 2003	+	+	n.c.	(+)	only indirect evidence of effectiveness
Hill and Doyon 1990	(+)	∅	not enough evidence	(+)	pos. and neg. results don't balance each other out
Jonas et al. 2000	+/(+)	(+)	significance not tenable after context analysis	(+)	n.c.
Kleijnen et al. 1991	+	(+)	mode of action of homeopathy not plausible	+	non-relevant rationale not shared
Linde et al. 1997	+	(+)/+	no clear statements about ill-nesses possible	+	arguments too restrictive
Linde and Jobst 1998	+	(+)	studies not relevant to practice	(+)	low clinical relevance
Linde and Mel-chart 1998	+/(+)	(+)	methodologi-cal short-comings	+	too much emphasis on internal validity not shared
Long 2001 ▼	+/(+)	(+)	not enough RCTs	(+)	n.c.

🔲 **Table 9.6** (continued)

Author, year	Result	Conclu-sion	Authors' rationale	Own conclusion	Reasons
Lüdtke 1999	+	(+)	'convincing indications of effectiveness'	(+)	n.c.
Lutz 1993	(+)	(+)	n.c.	(+)	n.c.
Smith 2001	∅	∅	n.c.	∅	n.c.
Vickers 2000	(+)	(+)	n.c.	(+)	n.c.
Walach 1997	(+)	(+)	n.c.	(+)	n.c.
Wiesenauer and Lüdtke 1996	+	+	n.c.	(+)	evaluation not independent as researcher = reviewer

Abbreviations:
n.c. no comment. No comment was necessary as evaluations did not differ.
+   significant result/ effectiveness very likely
(+) trend in favour of homeopathy
∅   no evidence for the effectiveness of homeopathy

9.5   Discussion and Conclusion

Results are discussed in detail in Chap. 13.

In the synthesis of results, 20 of 22 reviews found at least a trend in favour of homeopathy. We think that with five of the studies the results even clearly proved the effectiveness of a homeopathic intervention. Four reviews, including the highly controversial Linde study, examined the general effectiveness of homeopathy as a system. It must be pointed out that a follow-up study with higher external validity that examined how effective individualized classical homeopathy is also provided evidence of its effectiveness. One study investigated an acute clinical condition, postoperative ileus, where the use of various homeopathic remedies resulted in a statistically significant and clinically relevant effect.

In two (of 22) reviews no positive proof of effectiveness was found for the homeopathic treatment, but one of them focused on muscle soreness, a condition that is hardly practice-relevant, and probably not all studies were considered for its analysis (cf. Dean 1998). The other review was on homeopathic effectiveness in labour induction. It was based on only one clinical study with low internal and external validity, which showed no difference between verum and placebo group.

Conclusion after revision of reviews on homeopathy: on our three-tier evaluation scale ('likely, questionable, unlikely'), the effectiveness of homeopathy has to be rated as 'likely'. Despite this encouraging outcome, the following points need to be considered from the homeopathic point of view:

The large majority of studies mentioned in systematic and other reviews were carried out according to conventional medical standards as justification research, with a view to attaining outer recognition for homeopathy. Homeopathically speaking, most of these studies were conducted with inadequate, not practice-relevant methods, because their design ignored essential tenets of homeopathy, thus causing low model validity and a high risk of false-negative results.

One could say that the external validity was sacrificed in favour of internal validity and the research results are therefore of little value for actual homeopathic practice. They still serve the purpose of supplying fundamental evidence that (highly) potentized remedies applied with recognized methods can bring about a specific effect or efficacy (cf. Righetti 1999).

9.6   List of Excluded Studies with Reasons for Exclusion

Bol 1998. Neue Meta-Analyse zu randomisierten, kontrollierten Studien zur Homöopathie: die klinische Wirksamkeit der Homöopathie ist mehr als ein Placeboeffekt.
Not a systematic review

Coll 2001. Homeopathy in survivors of childhood sexual abuse
Not a systematic review

Dantas and Rampes 2000. Do homeopathic medicines provoke adverse effects? A systematic review.
See Chap. 11

Dean 1998. Out of step with the Lancet homeopathy meta-analysis: More objections than objectivity?
Comments on Ernst and Barnes 1998 (see there)

Demarque 1987. The development of proving methods since Hahnemann
Not a systematic review. Interesting aspects: single- and double-blind studies as well as crossover design and consideration of length of follow-up go back to 19th century homeopathic drug provings, before orthodox medicine had even begun to grasp the suggestive effect of pharmaceutical products. The difficulty of distinguishing which symptoms should be attributed to the homeopathic agent and which to the patient's essential disposition (Lamasson 1965) was already recognized then. It can therefore be assumed that the Materia Medica is based on thorough provings and considerations of a potential placebo effect. In drug provings one proceeds from the highest potency in descending order, until symptoms appear, followed by interval; next proving only when symptoms have subsided. Duration of follow-up: usually 8 weeks.

Ernst 1998. Are highly dilute homeopathic remedies placebos?
Re-analysis of Linde et al. 1997 (see there)

Ernst 2000. The usage of complementary therapies by dermatological patients: a systematic review
Not a systematic review on effectiveness, but on CAM use by dermatological patients. Seven studies found. Use (lifetime) between 35% and 69%. Most frequently homeopathy, phytotherapy and nutritional supplements. Usually satisfied with CAM. Reasons for use often dissatisfaction with conventional medicine. Use of CAM increased with duration and severity of disease. Results justify further intensive research into CAM.

Ernst and Resch 1996. Clinical trials of homeopathy: a re-analysis of a published review
Reanalysis of Kleijnen et al. 1991 (see there)

Ernst and Pittler 2000. Re-analysis of previous meta-analysis of clinical trials of homeopathy.
Comments on Linde et al. 1997 and Linde et al. 1999 (see there)

Fisher 1999. Delayed-onset muscle soreness in long-distance runners
Comment on Dean 1998 and Ernst and Barnes 1998 (see there)

Haidvogl et al. 1993. Homeopathic treatment of handicapped children
Not a systematic review. Several single case reports. Disabled children were allocated a homeo-pathic remedy via computer repertorisation after careful history-taking and constitutional type adjustment: 29 of 40 children showed improvement, 18 of them for all end points (end points were individually determined); seven children showed no improvement. Good response in case of organic brain damage, autism, hyperactivity, aggression, physical symptoms such as stutter and enuresis; poor results in case of social deprivation.

Jacobs et al. 2003. Homeopathy for childhood diarrhea: Combined results and meta-analysis from three randomized, controlled clinical trials
Not a systematic review, but meta-analysis of own three reviews, which each by itself had too low case numbers. Good: the Kaplan-Meier curve over time (proof of effectiveness based on Kiene!), but without variance bar. 'Normal' meta-analysis: effect size difference of ca. 0.66 days in favour of homeopathy (duration of diarrhoea with homeopathy 3.3, without 4.1 days), $p=0.008$. Conclusion: homeopathy is effective. Sufficient cases are necessary to 'lift the variance bar to ≥0'.

Jacobs 2002. Homeopathic research: fact or fantasy? – a review of the evidence
Not a systematic review, more like an anecdotal collection of evidence (many positive and a few negative studies, no systematic search strategy mentioned) or opinions. JAMA: there is no alternative medicine, only scientifically proven or unproven medicine. NEJM: homeopathy 'violates fundamental scientific laws'. Jacobs blames lack of funding ($ 60 m in 2001 for NHS, $ 3 m of that for placebo research, but hardly anything for homeopathy). Unfortunately, there really are not any often enough repeated studies on homeopathy [repetition of Linde's argument].

Jacobs et al. 1991. Alternative behandelingswijzen bij reumatische aandoeningen; een literatuuronderzoek
General overview of CAM. Not entirely clear whether a systematic research was really carried out. The data for homeopathy are not reproduced clearly enough to allow for own evaluation.

Jonas et al. 2003. A critical overview of homeopathy.
Not a systematic review of clinical studies, but general meta-review like those of Ernst, Linde and O'Meara, but without statement of search strategy. E reviews were considered in total. Description of study results. There is evidence of effectiveness, but not consistently: proven therapies should not be given up and substituted by homeopathy, but one should be open to further studies.

Jonas et al. 2001. A systematic review of the quality of homeopathic clinical trials
Not a systematic review on effectiveness, but on methodological quality. Research needed mainly to achieve higher replication rate of homeopathic studies (request for better reporting), request for higher reliability of measuring methods (e.g. the number of tonsillectomies is not

a reliable parameter, as the decision for or against tonsillectomy varies strongly among physicians).

Khan 2000. Clinical application of homeopathy podiatry as used at the Royal London Homeopathic Hospital (RLHH).

Not a systematic review, but a short report or poster. Homeopathic preparations are applied successfully for the topical treatment of foot or leg lesions such as hyperkeratoses or fungal infections.

Linde et al. 1994. Critical Review and Meta-analysis of Serial Agitated Dilutions in Experimental Toxicology

Systematic review of in-vitro and in-vivo animal and plant studies on serial agitated dilutions (SAD, as used in homeopathy for potentisation, e.g. for high potencies); inclusion criteria: in-vitro studies, in-vivo studies with animals or plants with experimentally induced intoxication, controlled studies, published in full text; own quality score; authors' information on strength of effect was checked with raw data. In 105 publications 135 experiments were found, mostly from bibliographical reference lists of PhD dissertations and review articles, 76% from France. Examination of arsenic, mercury, carbon tetrachloride, copper sulphate and various organic and inorganic substances in animal, plant, isolated organ or in-vitro models in various potencies (from low to high potentisation). Most studies were of poor quality (only 43% achieved more than 50% of possible maximum points). Only 26 studies met the meta-analysis criteria. The average protection rate beyond the control value was 19.7% (95 CI, 6.2–33.2). More studies are necessary.

Linde 1999. Gibt es gesicherte Therapien in der Homöopathie?

Not a systematic review, general overview of study situation. Rationale: From the scientific point of view, homeopathy is hardly plausible as a method. Therefore, more is expected, understandably, of a proof of effectiveness than with physiologically and pharmacologically 'more convincing' therapies. Collection of comparable studies on indications for which at least three studies are available:

Conclusion: No truly convincing proof of effectiveness has so far been adduced by independently reproduced, methodologically high-quality investigations.

Linde et al. 1998. Overviews and meta-analyses of controlled clinical trials of homeopathy

Not a systematic review; book contribution with contents of Linde review (Linde et al. 1997) and Clausius' PhD dissertation

Linde et al. 1999. Impact of study quality on outcome on placebo-controlled trials of homeopathy

Re-analysis of own data on Linde et al. 1997 (see there).

Linde and Willich 2003. How objective are systematic reviews? Differences between reviews on complementary medicine

Not a systematic review on effectiveness. Important methodological contribution! What are the reasons for the varying consideration of studies in systematic reviews with the same research question? Reviews on the same topic (indication, condition) include different numbers of stud-

◻ **Table 9.7** List of comparable homeopathic studies (Linde 1999)

Indication	Intervention	No. of studies	Result/comment
chronic headache	classical homeopathy	4	controversial/ some high-quality studies
diarrhoea in children	classical homeopathy	3	positive/ same reviewer
rheumatoid arthritis	classical homeopathy	3	controversial/ some of poor quality
hay fever	Galphimia glauca	7	positive/ same reviewer, high dropout rate
treatment for influenza	Oscillococcinum	4	positive/ two studies of questionable quality
muscle soreness	Rhus toxicodendron	4	positive trend/ same reviewer, quality questionable
muscle soreness	Arnica	4	negative
gastritis	Nux vomica	3	positive trend/ older study of questionable quality
muscle cramps	Cuprum	3	negative/ older studies of questionable quality

ies (2–17; 16–89); the reasons are: (a) time period of search (rare), (b) different inclusion criteria (population, duration of follow-up, English/other languages, databases, peer review).

Possible reasons for differing evaluations: different end points and end-point analyses (OR, combined p-value etc.), different meta-analysis models (random, fixed effects model, weighted sum of Z), different voting (in reporting (!), i.e. whether the author rates + or – , as well as in our own conclusion).

Lüdtke 2002. Statistical comments on a re-analysis of a previous meta-analysis of homeopathic RCTs

Comment on Ernst and Pittler 2000, Linde et al. 1997 (see there), and Linde et al. 1999.

Lüdtke and Bock 1995. Medikamentenprüfungen in der Praxis niedergelassener Ärzte – die Auswertung verschiedener Studien

Not a systematic review. Extensive description of the statistical analysis of the two Galphimia studies by Wiesenauer 1988 and 1989. Both studies with higher placebo effects. The 1989 study three-armed with placebo and not homeopathically diluted Galphimia compared with potentized Galphimia (the three-arm design makes little sense considering the patient number). Collaboration with many physicians in private practice with clearly differing motivation and cooperativeness, which means that a physician effect cannot be excluded. Bias probably mostly due to adjunct medication. Although the 1988 study did not formally show significance, an effectiveness of Galphimia was concluded. The same was not possible in the 1989 study, where data were possibly also confounded, leading to ten patients of one physician having to be excluded.

Lüdtke and Wiesenauer 1997. Eine Metaanalyse der homöopathischen Behandlung der Pollinosis mit Galphimia glauca
Not an original systematic review. Apparently double publication to Wiesenauer 1996.

McCarney et al. 2003. Homeopathy for dementia
Only the abstract was read. The authors conducted a search of the 'Specialized Register of the Cochrane Dementia and Cognitive Improvement Group' using the search terms alum*, homeop*, nat sulph* and natrium sulphate; further search in CISCOM, HomInform and AMED. Only RCTs with case number >20 were included. One study met inclusion criteria; after its full text had been read it was also excluded, so no data are available that are relevant to the research question.

Morrison et al. 2000. Methodological rigour and results of clinical trials of homeopathic remedies
Not a systematic review on effectiveness, but on methods: randomisation of studies used by Linde for his meta-analysis was evaluated (a) by a 'randomisation security panel' on the basis of the published study and (b) on the basis of the authors' answers to questions submitted to them. No correlation was found between results and treatment effects. It is interesting that, with the exception of two that were downgraded after receipt of the authors' answer and those where no answers were received, all were rated higher and often even achieved the maximum score of 8. The diagram is somewhat unintelligible, as it suggested that after the 'safe' evaluation a 'negative trend': high quality – poorer treatment effect would occur.

Poitevin 1988. Évaluation de l'homéopathie, axes généraux
Not a systematic review with systematic search and inclusion and exclusion criteria, rather an anecdotal collection of individual examination results, mainly from the laboratory, also including Beneviste experiments. Homeopathy works with animals and in the laboratory, indications that it works in human beings are also available, but the relevant studies need to be improved.

Righetti 1999. Homöopathie: Grundlagen, Anwendungsgebiete und mögliche Ansätze zu Forschungsstudien
Not a systematic review, but an overview of the research status in homeopathy established with the PEK project in mind, based on the previous, more extensive presentation by Righetti of 1988 'Research in homeopathy. Foundations, problems and results' as well as on the overview by Halter and Righetti 1999, with concise description of the fundamental problems with homeopathic research, the 'milestone study' of in-vitro, in-vivo and clinical research, as well as a detailed discussion of the possibilities of research methods that are suitable for homeopathy.

Scheen 1997. L'homéopathie peut-elle trouver sa légitimité dans les résultats "positif" d'une méta-analyse?
Not a systematic review, summary of Linde study. Does not think his meta-analysis alone is adequate proof of evidence for homeopathy. Also requests more comparisons to 'normal' medication.

Scofield 1984. Experimental research in homeopathy – a critical review
Semi-systematic review of homeopathic research in various fields. With regard to clinical experiments, Scofield quotes 15 studies starting from 1944 (Paterson with mustard gas) and going up to 1983 with partly good success rates for homeopathy. The conclusion, which also includes the non-clinical studies, was: 'Despite the great deal of experimental and clinical work there is only little scientific evidence to suggest that homeopathy is effective. This is because of the bad design, execution, reporting of failure to repeat experimental work and not necessarily because of the inefficacy of the system […]. Some of the experimental work already done suggests that homeopathy may be of value in the treatment and prevention of diseases in crops as well as animals and humans.'

Taylor et al. 2000. Randomized controlled trial of homeopathy versus placebo in perennial allergic rhinitis with overview of four trial series
Not a systematic review. Homeopathic medication for perennial allergic rhinitis. RCT with 50 patients, intervention: main allergen C30, with placebo control. No convincing effect in this trial, but after including three further trials (which were apparently not published?), the result turned positive for homeopathy after all.

Tveiten and Bruset 2002. Effect of Arnica D30 in marathon runners. Pooled results from two double-blind placebo controlled studies
Not a systematic review. Authors' own Oslo marathon results from 1990 and 1995 were pooled; 82 marathon runners were each given 5 verum or placebo pills morning and evening. Muscle pain immediately after running was less in the Arnica group (p=0.04) than with placebo but on peak with both groups, which is why the authors' conclusion of proven effectiveness is not entirely shared.

Van Wassenhoven 2002. Méta-analyse des travaux récents en clinique homéopathique
Not a systematic review, no systematic search with inclusion and exclusion criteria. He reports about recent meta-analyses on homeopathy, finds only seven systematic reviews, four of which are quantitative meta-analyses; discusses the more fundamental possibilities of effectiveness (evidence for hormesis etc.).

Walach 1992. Wissenschaftliche homöopathische Arzneimittelprüfung
Not a systematic review, but general overview of existing clinical and preclinical research with studies from 1954 onwards, e.g. Boyd: 15 years of preclinical experiments (wheat growth) up to D61(!) with positive results in favour of homeopathy, and relatively systematic literature from 1960 to 1984 including German and English studies and a few others up to 1986. No explicit inclusion or exclusion criteria. Twenty clinical studies. Negative/positive study ratio: 6/2. Of the negative ones only one was of good quality. Ratio of all studies (clinical and preclinical): ten neg/three pos, three equivalent. Few studies that meet the 'hard' criteria, but these few, together with the abundance of other findings, make it seem probable in a kind of cumulative, hermeneutic rationale that there are *sui generis* effects. Preclinical studies: Pelikan 1965: with 240 trials a significance level of 0.1%, Manswell 1975: dose-effect-curve in favour of potentisation. Possibility of side effects must not be ignored.

Wein 2002. Qualitätsaspekte klinischer Studien zur Homöopathie
Not a systematic review on effectiveness, but a very good methodological study. Its fundamental evaluation criteria for internal, external and model validity were mostly adopted by us.

Witt et al. 2000. Homeopathic treatment of human infertility – an overview
Abstract on systematic review. Twelve studies were identified, five were prospective clinical studies all conducted by the same team. (Apparently) three of them showed a positive trend (two observational studies and one matched-pair-analysis), two other studies were not completed due to recruitment problems.

Ziment and Tashkin 2000. Alternative medicine for allergy and asthma
Not a systematic review. Overview of several CAM methods; reports about Reilly's asthma and hay fever study and its discussion (editorial: Reilly's challenge, *Lancet* 1994, 344: 1585); also lists Kleijnen as a general source for the effectiveness of homeopathy in principle; more like a general overview of possible CAM therapies for physicians without CAM experience.

From the homeopathic point of view it must be concluded that there are studies among the excluded reviews and overviews which, with their extensive data and their positive results, are much more significant in favour of homeopathy than some of the work that has been included. The excluded titles with their wealth of positive evidence in favour of homeopathy therefore clearly support the thesis that homeopathy is effective.

9.7 References

Barnes J, Resch K-L, Ernst E (1997) Homeopathy for postoperative ileus? (A meta-analysis). J Clin Gastroenterol 25:628–633

Bauer CM, Weight L, Lambert MI (2002) The use of Arnica for the treatment of soft-tissue damage. S Afr J Physiother 58:34–40

Boissel JP, Cucherat M, Haugh M, Gauthier E (1996) Critical literature review on the effectiveness of homeopathy: overview of data from homeopathic medicine trials. In: Homeopathic Medicine Research Group. Report to the Commission of the European Union Communities, pp 196–210

Bol A (1998) Neue Meta-Analyse zu randomisierten, kontrollierten Studien in der Homöopathie: die klinische Wirksamkeit der Homöopathie ist mehr als ein Placeboeffekt. Homint R&D Newslett 1:10–3

Coll L (2001) Homeopathy in survivors of childhood sexual abuse. Homeopathy 91:3–9

Cucherat M, Haugh MC, Gooch M, Boissel JP (2000) Evidence of clinical efficacy of homeopathy. (A meta-analysis of clinical trials). Eur J Clin Pharmacol 56:27–33

Dantas F, Rampes H (2000) Do homeopathic medicines provoke adverse effects? A systematic review. Br Homeopathic J 89:35–38

Dean M (1998) Out of step with the Lancet homeopathy meta-analysis: more objections than objectivity? J Altern Complement Med 4:389–298

Demarque D (1987) The development of proving methods since Hahnemann. Br Homeopathic J 76:271–275

Ernst E (1998) Are highly dilute homeopathic remedies placebos? Perfusion 11:291–292

Ernst E (1999a) Homeopathic prophylaxis of headaches and migraine? A systematic review. J Pain Symptom Manage 18:353–357

Ernst E (1999b) Classical homeopathy versus conventional treatments: a systematic review. Perfusion 12:13–15

Ernst E (2000) The usage of complementary therapies by dermatological patients: a systematic review. Br J Dermatol 142:857–861

Ernst E (2002) A systematic review of systematic reviews of homeopathy. Br J Clin Pharmacol 54:577–582

Ernst E, Barnes J (1998) Are homeopathic remedies effective for delayed-onset muscle soreness? A systematic review of placebo-controlled trials. Perfusion 11:4–8

Ernst E, Pittler MH (1998) Efficacy of homeopathic Arnica; a systematic review of placebo-controlled clinical trials. Arch Surg 133:1187–1190

Ernst E, Pittler MH (2000) Re-analysis of previous meta-analysis of clinical trials of homeopathy (letter to the editors). J Clin Epidemiol 53:1188

Ernst E, Resch KL (1996) Clinical trials of homeopathy: a re-Analysis of a published review. Forschende Komplementärmedizin 3:85–90

Fisher P (1999) Delayed onset muscle soreness in long-distance runners. J Altern Complement Med 5:119

Glanville J, Sowden A (2001) Identification of the need for a review. In: Khan K, ter Riet G, Glanville J, Sowden A, Kleijnen J (eds). Undertaking Systematic Reviews of Research on Effectiveness. CRD Report Number 4 (2nd edn) York

Grabia S, Ernst E (2003) Homeopathic aggravations: a systematic review of randomized, placebo-controlled clinical trials. Homeopathy 92:92–98

Haidvogl M, Lehner E (1993) Homeopathic treatment of handicapped children: review of a series of 40 cases. Br Homeopathic J 82:227–236

Halter K, Righetti M (1998) Klassische Homöopathie (Teile 1–3) – Zum Nachweis von Wirksamkeit und Nutzen einer komplementärmedizinischen Methode. Schweiz Z GanzheitsMed 10:252–257, 343–346 and (1999) 11:1

Hill C, Doyon F (1990) Review of randomized trials of homeopathy. Rev Epidemiol Sante Publique 38:139–148

Jacobs J (2002) Homeopathic research: fact or fantasy? (A review of the evidence). Am J Homeopathic Med 95:26–32

Jacobs J, Jonas WB, Jimenez-Perez M, Crothers D (2003) Homeopathy for childhood diarrhea: combined results and meta-analysis from three randomized, controlled clinical trials. Pediatr Infect Dis J 22:229–234

Jacobs JWG, Rasker JJ, van Riel PLCM, Gribnau FWJ, van de Putte LBA (1991) Alternatieve behandelingswijzen bij reumatische aandoeningen; een literatuuronderzoek. Ned Tijdschr Geneeskd 135:317–322

Jonas WB, Anderson RL, Drawford DD, Lyons JS (2001) A systematic review of the quality of homeopathic clinical trials. BMC Complement Altern Med 1:1–12

Jonas WB, Kaptchuk Ted J, Linde K (2003) A critical overview of homeopathy. Ann Intern Med 138:393–399

Jonas WB, Linde K, Rampes H (2000) Homeopathy and rheumatic disease. Complement Altern Ther 26:117–123

Khan MT (2000) Clinical application of homeopathic podiatry as used at The Royal London Homeopathic Hospital (RLHH). Br Homeopathic J 89 [Suppl 1]:S53

Kleijnen J, Knipschild P, ter Riet G (1991) Clinical trials of homeopathy. BMJ 302:316–323

Linde K (1999) Are there proven therapies in homeopathy? [in German]. Internist (Berl) 40:1271–1274

Linde K, Clausius N, Ramirez G, Melchart D, Eitel F, Hedges LV, Jonas WB (1997) Are the clinical effects of homeopathy placebo effects? A meta-analysis of placebo-controlled trials. Lancet 350:834–843

Linde K, Clausius N, Ramirez G, Melchart D, Eitel F, Hedges LV, Jonas WB (1998) Overviews and meta-analyses of controlled clinical trials of homeopathy: in: Ernst E, Hahn EG (eds) Homeopathy. A critical appraisal. Butterworth-Heinemann, Oxford, pp 101–106

Linde K, Hondras M, Vickers A, ter Riet G, Melchart D (2001) Systematic reviews of complementary therapies – an annotated bibliography. Part 3: Homeopathy. BMC Complement Alternat Med 1:4. doi:10.1186/1472-6882-1-4

Linde K, Jobst K (2000) Homeopathy for asthma. The Cochrane Library (2). CD000353

Linde K, Jonas WB, Melchart D, Worku F, Wagner H, Eitel F (1994) Critical review and meta-analysis of serial agitated dilutions in experimental toxicology. Hum Exp Toxicol 13:481–492

Linde K, Melchart D (1998) Randomized controlled trials of individualized homeopathy: a state-of-the-art review. J Altern Complement Med 4:371–188

Linde K, Scholz M, Ramirez G, Clausius N, Melchart D, Jonas WB (1999) Impact of study quality on outcome in placebo-controlled trials of homeopathy. J Clin Epidemiol 52:631–636

Linde K, Willich SN (2003) How objective are systematic reviews? Differences between reviews on complementary medicine. J R Soc Med 96:17–22

Long LEE (2001) Homeopathic remedies for the treatment of osteoarthritis: a systematic review. Br Homeopathic J 90:37-43

Lüdtke R, Bock E (1995) Medikamentenprüfungen in der Praxis niedergelassener Ärzte – Die Auswertung verschiedener Studien. Institut für Medizinische Informationsverarbeitung der Universität Tübingen

Lüdtke R, Wilkens J (1999) Klinische Wirksamkeitsstudien zu Arnica in homöopathischen Zubereitungen. In: Albrecht H, Frühwald M (eds) Jahrbuch der Karl und Veronica Carstens-Stiftung, vol 5. KVC-Verlag, Essen, pp 97–112

Lüdtke R (2002) Statistical comments on a re-analysis of a previous meta-analysis of homeopathic RCTs. J Clin Epidemiol 55:103–104

Lüdtke R, Wiesenauer M (1997) Eine Metaanalyse der homöopathischen Behandlung der Pollinosis mit Galphimia glauca. Wien Med Wochenschr 147:323–327

Lutz, C (1993) Quantitative Meta-Analyse empirischer Ergebnisse der Homöopathieforschung. Diplomarbeit, Psychologisches Institut, Albert-Ludwigs-Universität, Freiburg

McCarney R, Warner J, Fisher P, van Haselen R (2003) Homeopathy for dementia. The Cochrane Library (2) CD003803

Morrison B, Lilford RJ, Ernst E (2000) Methodological rigour and results of clinical trials of homeopathic remedies. Perfusion 13:132–138

O'Meara S, Wilson P, Bridle C, Kleijnen J (2003) Effectiveness of homeopathy: a systematic review of systematic reviews. Quality Safety Health 11:189–194

Poitevin B (1988) Evaluation de l`homeopathe, axes generaux. Homeopathie française 76:93

Righetti M (1988) Forschung in der Homöopathie. Grundlagen, Problematik und Ergebnisse. Burgdorf, Göttingen

Righetti M (1999) Homöopathie: Grundlagen, Anwendungsgebiete und mögliche Ansätze zu Forschungsstudien. available at: http://www.homeodoctor.ch/Righetti.htm

Scheen AJ (1997) L'homéopathie peut-elle trouver sa légitimité dans les résultats "positifs" d'une méta-analyse? Rev Med Liege 52:694–697

Scofield AM (1984) Experimental research in homeopathy – a critical review. Br Homeopathic J 73:161–180 and 211–226

Smith CA (2001) Homeopathy for induction of labour. The Cochrane Library 4:1-11

Taylor MA, Reilly D, Llewellyn-Jones RH, McSharry Ch, Aitchison TC (2000) Randomized controlled trial of homeopathy versus placebo in perennial allergic rhinitis with overview of four trial series. BMJ 321:471–476

Tveiten D, Bruset S (2003) Effect of Arnica D30 in marathon runners. Pooled results from two double-blind placebo controlled studies. Homeopathy 92:187–189

van Wassenhoven M (2002) Meta-analyse des travaux recents en clinique homeopathique. (Revue Belge D`Homeopathie). available at: http://www.entretiens-internationaux.mc/wwfdeux.htm

Vickers A, Smith CA (2000) Homeopathic Oscillococcinum for preventing and treating influenza and influenza-like syndromes. The Cochrane Library (1):CD001957

Walach H (1997)Unspezifische Therapie-Effekte – Das Beispiel Homöopathie. Habilitationsschrift Psychologisches Institut, Albert-Ludwigs-Universität Freiburg

Walach H (1992) Wissenschaftliche homöopathische Arzneimittelprüfung. Doppelblinde Crossover-Studie einer homöopathischen Hochpotenz gegen Placebo. Haug, Heidelberg

Wein C (2002) Qualitätsaspekte klinischer Studien zur Homöopathie. KVC-Verlag, Essen

Wiesenauer M, Lüdtke R (1996) A meta-analysis of the homeopathic treatment of pollinosis with Galphimia glauca. Forschende Komplementärmedizin 3:230–234

Witt C, Müller E, Linde K, Willich SN (2000) Homeopathic treatment of human infertility – an overview. Reprod Domestic Animals 35:17

Ziment I, Tashkin DP (2000) Alternative medicine for allergy and asthma. J Allergy Clin Immunol 106:603–614

Reactions)

10

Clinical Studies on the Effectiveness of Homeopathy for URTI/A (Upper Respiratory Tract Infections and Allergic Reactions)

Stefanie Maxion Bergemann, Gudrun Bornhöft, Denise Bloch, Christina Vogt-Frank, Marco Righetti, André Thurneysen

10.1   Selection of Indication

This HTA uses systematic surveys, clinical studies and single case reports to research the effectiveness of homeopathic methods of treatment. It needs clinical studies on relevant indications for which sufficient RCTs, non-randomized prospective controlled and uncontrolled trials are available, as well as high-quality case studies.

The clinical indication should be relevant to the practical significance of the selected domain and to its applicability in homeopathy.

Applicability here means that it has to be suited to the specific approach of classical homeopathy, where symptoms are not categorized in terms of a diagnosis as in conventional medicine, but the individual symptoms in their entirety are seen as corresponding to a drug picture.

Local symptoms such as 'redness, pounding pain' in association with the general symptoms 'moist-sweaty, shivery, restless to anxious' can suggest otitis media or tonsillitis or a skin infection. For all three diagnoses the symptoms match the drug picture of belladonna. Even otitides of identical infectiology which manifest in different kinds of pain and overall symptoms correspond to different homeopathic remedies. This means that treatment is determined not by the diagnosis, but by the drug picture (Walach 1996).

For the investigation of the 'real-world' effectiveness of homeopathy, studies are therefore needed that describe indications which are as relevant to clinical practice as to homeopathy. Haidvogl (1993) considers that the best study designs for this purpose are those that focus on the distinct local symptoms of well-defined indications.

Examination of the study material available in systematic reviews which reflect the study situation as from 1975 (e.g. Linde et al. 1997) showed that 'upper respiratory tract infections' (URTI) and 'allergic reactions' (A) meet these criteria and that sufficient studies were available for evaluation. URTI/A are, in all age and population groups, among the most frequent reasons for seeking medical help and they come with well-definable, objective and subjective symptoms that can be drawn on for evaluating the success of the treatment. As acute conditions URTI/A provide, in principle, a clear time frame which is suitable for trials, the possibility to assess recurrence and to differentiate the transition to the chronic stage should the situation arise (e.g. sinusitis).

URTI/A include the following complaints:
- acute rhinitis
- allergic rhinitis
- allergic asthma
- sinusitis
- adenoid vegetations
- pharyngitis and tonsillitis
- influenza-like infection
- otitis media

10.2   Outcome of Literature Search

Forty-one studies were found in total for the indication 'upper respiratory tract infections/allergic reactions' (URTI/A). Three studies were double publications to studies that were already included. Six other articles were excluded from further evaluation after their full text had been read because they did not deal with URTI/A (for reasons for exclusion see ☐ Table 10.5). Three studies could not be obtained in the time available (Burke et al. 1991; Weiser and Clasen 1994 and 1995); the same was the case with two comprehensive dissertations on purulent angina (Fournier 1979; Bauhof 1982; quoted from Righetti 1988).

The systematic search in online libraries produced 11 studies; another 16 studies were found by systematically searching the bibliographical references of the former studies, and two more studies were found through personal contacts.

The following information is based entirely on 29 evaluated studies (see ■ Tables 10.1–10.3).

We experienced one fundamental problem: despite a thorough web search in the indexed literature, inspection of bibliographical reference lists of homeopathic studies and personal contacts, only some of the actually existing studies were found, which means that our assessment – just like other similar studies – is not complete.

Clinical studies on URTI/A: description and results of individual studies

The studies were conducted in different countries: Germany (15 studies), UK (8), one study each in France, Switzerland, USA, the Netherlands and Norway. One study had centres in various countries.

The largest study examined 1479 patients, while the smallest 'study' is a single case report. In all, the studies contain results from 5062 patients.

The individual indications were spread across the studies as follows: otitis media (6 studies), allergic rhinitis (5), influenza-like infection (4), asthma (4), URTI/A without further differentiation (3), sinusitis (2), adenoid vegetations (1), infectious mononucleosis (1), cough (1), allergic asthma (1) and tonsillitis (1).

■ **Studies on URTI/A, general:**

The following section briefly introduces the individual indications, their habitual treatment in conventional medicine and the corresponding homeopathy studies with their results.

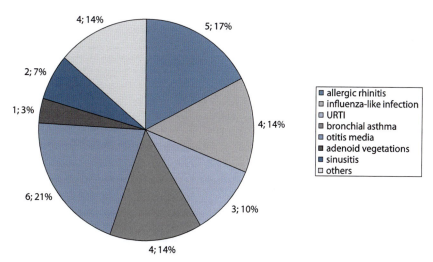

■ **Fig. 10.1** Number and proportion (*n*; %) of publications on individual URTI/A indications

■■ **Studies:**

1. de Lange de Klerk (1994). Effect of homeopathic medicines on daily burden of symptoms in children with recurrent upper respiratory tract infection

The randomized, placebo-controlled double-blind study measured the impact of individualized homeopathic therapy on a daily assessed symptom score (with four parameters), on the number of antibiotic treatments and on the number of adenoidectomies and tonsillectomies in 170 children. The mean daily symptom score was 2.61 in the placebo group and 2.21 in the treatment group (difference 0.41, 95% CI, -0.02–0.83). In both groups the use of antibiotics was greatly reduced compared with the previous year. The percentage of children who had adenoidectomies (16%; 8/50) was lower in the homeopathically treated group than in the placebo group (21%; 9/42). For children who had tonsillectomies the results were the same in both groups. The authors conclude that individualized homeopathic treatment has an effect, if a small one, on URTI/A (EBM evidence grade[1] 1b).

2. Herzberger and Weiser (1997) Homöopathische Behandlung von Infekten unterschiedlicher Genese – eine Anwendungsbeobachtung

The prospective, multi-centre observational study (without a control group) assessed the application, effectiveness and tolerability of Engystol® in combination with other therapies for URTI/A based on data retrieved from 1479 cases treated by 154 physicians. The success of the treatment was measured based on the time when the first signs of improvement occurred and on the global evaluation of the therapy results obtained using a five-tier scale.

About half of the patients reported noticeable improvement of symptoms within 1–4 days; only 6% of patients registered no improvement. The point in time of subjective improvement setting in depended, among other things, on the symptom picture: for patients suffering from influenza or febrile infections the result was very good to good in almost 90% of the cases. For the prophylactic use of Engystol® to strengthen the body's defences the result was described as 'good' to 'very good' by 85%. The same success rates were reported for patients who used medicinal and physical adjuvant therapies (870 of 1479 patients).

Adverse drug effects were registered in four cases, three of which were not associated with the use of Engystol®. The tolerability of the homeopathic treatment, described as 'excellent' to 'good' by 97%, was also observed in combination with other therapies (EBM evidence grade 3).

3. Riley et al. (2001). Homeopathic and conventional medicine: an outcomes study comparing effectiveness in a primary care setting.

The multi-centre controlled trial examined the effectiveness of homeopathic compared with conventional medical treatment in 456 patients suffering from respiratory tract disorders. A statistically significant clinical and subjective improvement of the complaints was registered after 14 days in 82.6% of patients in the homeopathy group and in 68% of the conventionally treated group ($p = 0.0058$). Side effects were documented in 7.8% of the homeopathy group and in 22.3% of the conventionally treated group. The authors concluded a clear superiority of homeopathy over conventional treatment in the cases examined (EBM evidence grade 2b).

■   **Acute and allergic rhinitis**

Acute rhinitis usually occurs in stages: the catarrhal stage begins with a tickling sensation and sneezing followed by watery secretion and nasal obstruction and hyposmia. After a few days the

---

1   For evidence grading see p. 29

mucous discharge stage sets in with red, swollen mucosa. Often the skin around the nostrils is affected due to the sharpness of the secretion and the mechanical strain of frequently blowing the nose.

Rhinitis is mostly caused by viruses, e.g. adenoviruses, which are spread by airborne droplets. Rhinitis also occurs concomitantly, with measles for instance.

Conventional treatment includes nasal decongestant drops as well as antipyretic and analgesic drugs. They do not usually curtail the duration of the disease, but they alleviate the symptoms.

Allergic rhinitis – also known as hay fever or pollinosis – has the catarrhal appearance of rhinitis with endonasal itching, sneezing attacks and clear secretion, often accompanied by strong burning and watering of the eyes and tiredness. The incidence of seasonal allergic rhinitis depends on the pollen count of the respective allergens; perennial rhinitis is caused mostly by dust, mould, animal hair or allergens at the workplace. The medical history, skin prick testing and serological detection of specific antibodies can identify the agents that cause it.

Treatment includes the avoidance and/or reduction of allergens, if necessary also cromoglicic acid, and antihistamines, as well as corticoid sprays. If the allergens are known, desensitisation can also be attempted.

■■ Studies:

4. Aabel (2000). No beneficial effect of isopathic prophylactic treatment for birch pollen. RCT of Betula C 30.

The randomized double-blind study examined the prophylactic effect of Betula C30 in comparison to placebo over 4 weeks in 73 participants with pollen allergy who had to complete a daily visual analogue scale (VAS) for the different symptoms. The figures were higher (i.e. a worse result) for the homeopathic treatment group during the 3 days of observation, and the use of 'rescue' medication was higher compared with the placebo group. It has to be pointed out that the prophylactic use of homeopathic treatment does not comply with homeopathic principles, a fact which considerably reduces the external validity of the trial. The authors also mention that weather conditions were particularly bad at the time of the trial and exposure to allergens consequently low compared with previous years, a circumstance which further restricts the usability of the results (EBM evidence grade 1b).

5. Reilly and Taylor (1985). Potent placebo or potency?

The randomized model study describes the results of a comparison between homeopathic treatment and placebo in 39 hay-fever sufferers; based on the symptom score (consisting of six symptoms), a trend in favour of homeopathy is demonstrated (EBM evidence grade 1b).

6. Reilly et al. (1986). Is homeopathy a placebo response? Controlled trial of homeopathic potency, with pollen in hay fever as model

The randomized double-blind trial examined the effect of homeopathic potencies ('mixed grass pollen 30c') against placebo in 144 hay-fever sufferers. The results showed significant improvement of a global symptom score (assessed via visual analogue scale: VAS), in the physician's estimation (mean VAS change: homeopathically treated group: –27.7 mm, SD 34.1; placebo group: –12.2 mm, SD 40.5) as well as in the patient's (mean VAS change: homeopathy group: –17.2 mm, SD 28.8; placebo group: –2.6 mm, SD 33.6). Antihistamine use was significantly lower in the homeopathic group (average number of tablets 11.2, SD: 13.5) compared with the placebo group (average number of tablets 19.7, SD: 18.6) (EBM evidence grade 1b).

To start with, an increased symptom aggravation was observed in the homeopathically treated group compared with the placebo group. The authors interpreted these as initial aggravations, which are a well-known phenomenon in homeopathy and indicate effectiveness.

7. Taylor et al. (2000). Randomized controlled trial of homeopathy versus placebo on perennial allergic rhinitis with overview of four trial series

The randomized, placebo-controlled, double-blind trial with 50 patients suffering from allergic rhinitis showed significant improvement of the nasal airflow for the homeopathically treated group (30c preparation of the allergen) compared with the placebo group (the overall improvement of nasal airflow was 21% in the homeopathically treated group. The improvement in the placebo group was only 2%, which corresponds to $p = 0.0001$ in the comparison of groups). Both groups improved the symptom scores, with a trend for the homeopathically treated group (difference to baseline: homeopathy group: -5.0; SD: 3.3; placebo group: -4; SD: -9.8–7.8; difference not significant). More initial aggravations were observed in the homeopathically treated group than in the placebo group: 7 vs. 2 (corresponding to 39% vs. 7%, $p = 0.0007$), but they were all remedied by day 16 (EBM evidence grade 1b).

8. Wiesenauer and Gaus (1985). Double-blind trial comparing the effectiveness of the homeopathic preparation Galphimia potentization D6, Galphimia dilution 10-6 and placebo on pollinosis

The controlled randomized double-blind trial with 164 hay-fever patients compared the effectiveness of Galphimia D6 with that of a non-homeopathic 10^{-6} dilution and placebo (three-arm trial) by observing nose and eye symptoms on a 4-point-scale (1: symptom-free to 4: no improvement) at two subsequent GP consultations that were a fortnight apart.

At the first consultation improvement or freedom from eye symptoms were reported for 34/48 patients (71%) in the Galphimia D6 group, for 27/55 (49%) in the Galphimia 10^{-6} group and 30/50 (60%) in the placebo group. Improvement or freedom from nasal symptoms was registered by 30/50 patients (60%) in the Galphimia D6 group, 22/55 (40%) in the Galphimia 10^{-6} group and 24/50 (41%) in the placebo group. At the second consultation the results showed a similar trend for Galphimia D6. Adverse effects were not reported. Although no statistical significance was achieved, the group treated with Galphimia D6 showed a positive trend (EBM evidence grade 1b).

The trial also provides evidence of the pharmacodynamic differences between the preparations gained from the same original substance, depending on whether they were simply diluted or homeopathically potentized.

- **Sinusitis**

Acute sinusitis usually develops from rhinitis when the infection spreads to the mucous membrane of the sinuses, primarily affecting the maxillary and ethmoid, more rarely the frontal sinuses (very rarely the sphenoid sinuses). Combination with an allergic genesis is also possible.

Characteristic symptoms are pressure and pain in the maxillary sinuses with mucoid to dry discharge. Headaches caused by bending, applying pressure and nose-blowing are typical too. Fever and general malaise can accompany the local symptoms and exacerbate the infection. The danger of complications such as meningitis arises when the infection is spread within the neighbourhood.

Physical examination can cause headache above the affected sinuses; maxillary tooth ache is also common. Rhinoscopy discloses mucosal swelling in the medial nasal passage and purulent discharge. Ultrasound and X-ray imaging can reveal congestion of the normally air-filled cavities.

Primary treatment is with decongestants and substances that help loosen secretions, followed by inhalations, heat application and antipyretic and analgesic drugs. Antibiotics are used in advanced conditions and for complications.

The transition to chronic sinusitis is seamless if the condition persists or recurs more than three times per year.

■■ Studies:

9. Weber et al. (2002). A non-randomized pilot study to compare complementary and conventional treatments of acute sinusitis

The multi-centre controlled trial including 63 patients with acute sinusitis compared the effectiveness of homeopathic (Cinnabaris C3 was specified, but individual treatment was also permitted) and conventional treatment. In the physician evaluation the treatment success showed an advantage of 1.8 score points for the conventional group; in the patient evaluation the homeopathically treated group was slightly more successful, with 0.2 score points. This applies also to the change in life-quality score (HCG questionnaire) by 0.8 points. The results were adjusted for propensity score and centre effects. For all comparisons p was above 0.3, which means that there were no noticeable differences between conventional and homeopathic treatment.

The information regarding the use of medication in both groups was also of interest: in the conventional group 32/33 patients were given antibiotics, 32/33 sympathomimetics and 5/33 analgesics, while these drugs were not at all used in the homeopathic group: Additional medication there was Sinupret® in 26/30 cases (only one patient in the conventional group), and 20/30 patients (only 12 in the conventional group) applied inhalations.

The authors conclude that the effectiveness is at least comparable in both groups, while pointing out that the groups were not homogeneous and comparability was therefore restricted. It would need 400 patients to prove therapeutic equivalence (EBM evidence grade 2a).

10. Wiesenauer et al. (1989). Efficiency of homeopathic drug combinations for the treatment of sinusitis

The randomized double-blind trial with 47 physicians and 152 patients suffering from acute sinusitis examined the therapeutic effect of three homeopathic combinations and placebo on clinical symptoms. In all four groups acute sinusitis improved in 81% of the patients and chronic sinusitis in 67%, a result that is comparable to the rates published for conventional therapies. There was no noticeable difference between the groups and the placebo group (EBM evidence grade 1b). None of the groups reported adverse drug effects.

The authors compared their study results with published reports on spontaneous resolution and the successful use of antibiotics and conclude similar success rates for all the therapies named.

All in all, the authors evaluated the therapies available as insufficient and request that more practice-relevant conditions such as sinusitis find stronger consideration and that GPs become more involved in the research.

■ Pharyngitis and tonsillitis

Acute pharyngitis often occurs as part of an upper respiratory tract infection: a sore throat and discomfort when swallowing, a 'hot-potato' voice, and occasional dryness are characteristic symptoms. It frequently comes with pain that radiates into the ears, painful swollen lymph nodes and sometimes fever.

Pharynx inspection discloses reddened, often oedematous mucosa at the back of the throat; the tonsils can be equally red and swollen.

Suppurative tonsils usually suggest a bacterial infection called 'angina tonsillaris' which can present with confluent suppuration, massive swelling and abscesses that terminate in perforation. The raspberry tongue and exanthema are typical for scarlet fever caused by group A β-haemolytic streptococci.

With mononucleosis caused by the Epstein-Barr virus pseudo-membranes cover the tonsils; it is often not easy to clinically distinguish it from ordinary tonsillitis. Complications can arise if organs are affected (cervical lymph node swelling, splenomegaly and hepatomegaly).

The symptoms of pharyngitis can be alleviated by gargling with salt water or astringents or by taking analgesic or antipyretic drugs, vitamin C etc.

With angina, antibiotics are the remedy of choice. It is up to the treating physician to decide when to begin treatment.

Once the presence of β-haemolytic streptococci has been confirmed, antibiotics are the standard therapy to avoid complications such as rheumatic fever (RF) and poststreptococcal glomerulonephritis (GN).

▪▪ Studies:

11. Nusche (1998). Homöopathie oder Penicillin bei Mandelentzündung – eine prospektive klinische Studie.
In this controlled, prospective trial classical homeopathic treatment of 51 children with tonsillitis was compared with conventional penicillin treatment. The acute disease course (improvement in the first 48 h) was assessed by means of symptom scoring. The result was significantly positive for the control. There was also a noticeable trend for more purulent complications (especially otitis media) in the homeopathically treated group. The author does not exclude the basic effectiveness of homeopathic treatment, but she underlines the necessity to revise the homeopathic treatment for this disorder (EBM evidence grade 2a).

12. Bahemann (2002). Kalium bromatum bei infektiöser Mononukleose
Single-case documentation describing the successful treatment of a patient with infectious mononucleosis. The simultaneousness of treatment and improvement of symptoms in the patient can be seen as an indication for the effectiveness of the therapy. (EBM evidence grade 4).

▪ Influenza-like infection, bronchitis

Influenza-like infection is the name for a complex of conditions which presents with a combination of rhinitis, febrile pharyngitis, general tiredness and malaise. Coughing is, after vertebral column disorders, the second most common reason for seeing a doctor.

In the early stages it is difficult to distinguish from 'real influenza', which is caused by endemic spreading of the influenza viruses A and B.

Treatment is as above. Symptoms can be alleviated and the duration curtailed with amantadine or the new peroral neuraminidase inhibitors.

■ ■ **Studies: influenza-like infection**

13. Ferley et al. (1989). A controlled evaluation of a homeopathic preparation in the treatment of influenza-like symptoms

For this controlled, randomized, double-blind trial 487 patients with influenza-like infections were treated homeopathically in comparison to placebo. Recovery in the first 48 h (reduction of rectal temperature to 37.5°C and the complete disappearance of all assessed symptoms) was observed in 17.1% of the verum group and in 10.3% of the placebo group (p=0.03). Further analyses revealed a significant advantage in the homeopathic group with patients aged 12–29 for recovery within 48 h, the same for patients with light to medium severe symptoms (p <0.01 in each case). The authors conclude possible effectiveness of the homeopathic treatment but request further trials with strict design specification (EBM evidence grade 1b).

14. Gassinger et al. (1981). Klinische Prüfung zum Nachweis der Wirksamkeit von Eupatorium perfoliatum D2 bei grippalen Infekten

In a randomized controlled clinical trial with 53 patients suffering from influenza-like infections the effect of acetylsalicylic acid and Eupatorium perfoliatum D2 on subjective symptoms and clinical findings on days 1, 4 and 10 of the treatment were compared. No significant differences were found with regard to either symptoms, febrile course or lab results (EBM evidence grade 1b).

15. Maiwald et al. (1988). Therapie des grippalen Infektes mit einem homöopathischen Kombinationspräparat im Vergleich zu Acetylsalicylsäure

In a monocentric controlled, randomized trial on 170 soldiers with influenza-like infections the effectiveness of a homeopathic combination (Grip-Heel®) and acetylsalicylic acid (ASS) were compared. Measurement of clinical findings and subjective complaints on days 4 and 10 of the treatment and the length of inability to work showed no significant difference. Adverse effects were observed for three patients in the homeopathy group and for seven patients in the ASS group. A more detailed description was not supplied. The products can therefore be seen as comparably effective for influenza-like infections (EBM evidence grade 1b).

16. Papp and Schuback (1998). Oscillococcinum® in patients with influenza-like symptoms

A randomized, controlled, double-blind trial that examined the effectiveness of Oscillococcinum® against placebo in 372 patients with influenza-like infections. Symptom relief (score of 14 symptoms) within the first 48 h and the duration of symptoms were measured. In the homeopathically treated group 19.2% of patients were symptom-free after 48 s compared with only 15% in the control group, which means that, with p=0.0028, the result for the homeopathy group is statistically significant (EBM evidence grade 1b).

■ ■ **Cough studies**

17. Rabe (2001). Treatment of cough of different genesis with a modern homeopathic preparation

Prospective, uncontrolled cohort study with 339 cough patients (mostly acute bronchitis) to examine the effectiveness and tolerability of Husteel®; 71 physicians of various specialisations took part in the trial. The only conditions were that no other cough medicines be used and that Husteel® be used for a maximum period of 6 weeks. General improvement of the five clinical symptoms evaluated was observed in 45% of the patients within the first 3 treatment days. The calculated clinical score improved in the 19 days of observation from 1.5 points (moderate to poor) to 2.9 points (good). The treatment success was rated 'very good' or 'good' by the physicians for 96% of the patients and confirmed by 95% of the patients. Where Husteel® was the only treatment applied (other cough medicines were not permitted, but analgesic and antirheumatic drugs, antibiotics and physical measures such as inhalations could be used) 98% of physicians and patients documented the same evaluation. The physicians rated the overall tolerability 'very good' or 'good' in all cases.

The fact that the data did not state the standard deviation or confidence interval of the symptom scores for the group reduces the validity of the publication (EBM evidence grade 3).

- ### Syringitis (secretory otitis media or 'glue ear') and otitis media

Syringitis is caused by serous or mucoid effusion in the middle ear resulting from obstructed ventilation or drainage in the Eustachian tubes following catarrhal disease of the nasopharyngeal area, adenoid vegetations, allergies and other obstructive disorders. Symptoms include conductive hearing loss and sometimes a sense of pressure in the ear. Children up to the age of 6 years often have delayed speech development due to impaired hearing.

Otoscopy can disclose an often shiny, amber-coloured liquid behind the tympanic membrane; if the condition persists the tympanic membrane is often retracted. The tympanogram is flat and shows little movement of the eardrum; the pure tone audiogram reveals conductive hearing loss.

Treatment generally includes decongestant nasal drops, gum to encourage chewing[2]* and if necessary treatment of the underlying disease. If complaints persist for over 6 weeks und the condition turns chronic, paracentesis or grommet insertion might be indicated.

Acute otitis media is characterized by strong ear ache, loss of hearing, often fever with general malaise. Children between the ages of 6 months and 3 years are most frequently affected; 75–95% of children have had at least one, 30% even three or more episodes (Kruse 2004).

Otoscopy typically shows redness and bulging (initially only of the posterior, inferior quadrant), in some cases also spontaneous perforation of the eardrum. Tympanometry and a hearing test, in rare cases also an X-ray scan (e.g. in case of suspected mastoiditis) complete the diagnostic procedure.

The most common complications with acute otitis are persistent conductive hearing loss, frequent recurrence and chronicity, and impaired hearing, as well as spreading of the infection to adjacent areas leading to mastoiditis, meningitis or a brain abscess.

Recommended treatment includes decongestant nasal drops, antipyretics, analgesics and antibiotics.

- ## Studies:

18. Frei & Turneysen (2001). Homeopathy in acute otitis media in children: treatment effect or spontaneous resolution?

Cohort study to examine effectiveness of individualized homeopathic treatment in 230 children with otitis media. Pain relief occurred in 39% of patients within 6 h and in another 33% within 12 h. The authors compared the result with publications for placebo and concluded a resolution rate that was 2.4 times higher for the homeopathically treated children. No complications were observed. Based on information from Switzerland, the authors calculated the treatment costs and found them to be 14% lower for homeopathically treated patients than in a comparable population receiving conventional medical treatment (antibiotics, nasal spray). (EBM evidence grade 3)

---

2   *improves Eustachian tube ventilation (Gesenhues, Zicke; Praxisleitfäden Allgemeinmedizin, 1998)

19. Friese (1994). Therapie der akuten Mittelohrentzündung bei Kindern – Mit homöo-pathischen Mitteln gut behandelbar
The prospective cohort study involved 30 children with otitis media; 29 of the children received individualized homeopathic treatment, partly also physical therapies, and one child had anti-biotics in addition. The success rate was assessed on the basis of tympanogram, otoscopy (tym-panic membrane finding) and clinical symptoms. After an average of 34 days, seven of the 29 patients showed no TM abnormality (NAD[3]), while 14 patients still had signs of infection. After 2 weeks examination results came out negative for 90% of the patients. The number of patients who failed to attend follow-up examinations reduces the validity of the results. The author concludes from the study results that the success of homeopathic treatment is at least equivalent to that of conventional treatment with antibiotics (EBM evidence grade 3).

20. Friese et al. (1997c). The homeopathic treatment of otitis media in children – comparisons with conventional therapy
The prospective, controlled, non-randomized trial involving 131 children suffering from otitis media compared classical homeopathic with conventional medical treatment (including anti-biotics). Pain persisted for 2 days (median) in the homeopathically treated group and for 3 days in the conventionally treated group (p=0.1186). Treatment lasted 4 days in the homeopathy group and 10 days in the allopathy group (due to specified antibiotics course). Freedom from recurrence after 1 year was 70.7% in the homeopathically treated group and 56.5% in the con-ventionally treated group (p not given). Five of 103 children in the homeopathically treated group received antibiotics in addition compared with 23 of 28 children in the conventionally treated group. No severe side effects were reported; in the conventionally treated group mild gastrointestinal symptoms were observed (no exact figure stated). The authors conclude from the results that homeopathic treatment of otitis media constitutes a very good and safe alterna-tive to conventional antibiotic treatment (EBM evidence grade 2a).

21. Harrison et al. (1999). A randomized comparison of homeopathic and standard care for the treatment of glue ear in children
The non-blinded, randomized, controlled study was the pilot project for research into whether homeopathic therapy – compared with the usual allopathic treatment – can favourably influ-ence a hearing loss of more than 20 dB following acute otitis media within 12 months (i.e. res-toration to less than 20 dB). Thirty-two children were examined in total. Comparison of results after 12 months showed hearing loss of less than 20 dB for a larger percentage of the homeo-pathically treated children than of those conventionally treated (64% vs. 56%), although this difference did not reach statistical significance (95% CI for the difference between means of –25% and 42%). Antibiotics consumption and referral to specialists were also lower in the homeopathic group (not statistically significant); (EBM evidence grade 1b).

22. Jacobs et al. (2001a). Homeopathic treatment of acute otitis media in children: a pre-liminary randomized placebo-controlled trial
The trial was conducted as a randomized, double-blind controlled pilot study in a private paediatric surgery in Seattle to compare the effectiveness of homeopathic treatment with pla-cebo. Outcome parameters were the number of treatment failures after 5 days and 2 and 6 weeks. In addition, clinical symptoms and ear effusion were recorded in patient diaries.

---

3   NAD – no abnormality detected

The result showed fewer treatment failures in the homeopathically treated group, although the difference was not statistically significant. The assessment of symptoms in diaries, in contrast, showed a significant advantage for the homeopathic treatment. As this was a pilot study with a small case number, the result would have to be confirmed by a larger trial (243 children per group minimum, here 75 children in total).

The study shows that individualized homeopathic therapy can also be assessed and adequately applied within an RCT context. (EBM evidence grade 1b).

23. Mössinger (1985). Zur Behandlung der Otitis media mit Pulsatilla

The controlled, double-blind study examined the effectiveness of pulsatilla against placebo in 28 children with otitis media. The results showed no difference for the temperature development in the two groups, but the final physician evaluation presented a significant difference in favour of the pulsatilla group ($p<0.05$). The validity of the evaluation is restricted due to the fact that the information about blinding is ambiguous and also because of the small group size for both treatment methods (EBM evidence grade 1b).

▪ Adenoid vegetations

Enlarged adenoids are hyperplastic pharyngeal tonsils found predominantly in children due to their particularly active immune system (usually up to the age of 10) (Friese 1997).

Obstruction of the nasopharynx leads to open-mouth breathing, snoring at night and dry mucosa with sore throat in the morning. As a result, infections of the upper respiratory tract, secretory otitis media with recurring otitides, and hearing and speech impairment, as well as diminished concentration due to disturbed sleep, occur frequently. The condition gave rise to the expression 'adenoid facies' which refers to the fact that the open-mouthed and often dull appearance of the child makes him or her look less intelligent. Visualisation and epipharyngoscopy disclose large, mostly deeply grooved pharyngeal tonsils.

The treatment of choice addresses concomitant conditions and sequelae or consists in surgical removal if indicated due to complications.

▪▪ Studies:

24. Friese et al. (2001). Results of RCT on homeopathic treatment of adenoid vegetations

In a monocentric, prospective, randomized trial the effectiveness of homeopathic treatment (mostly individualized) was compared with that of placebo in 97 children with adenoid vegetation and existing indication for surgery. Evaluation was based on tympanoscopy, tympanometry, audiometry and revision of the surgery indication; 70.7% of the placebo-group children and 78.1% of the homeopathically treated group no longer needed surgery ($p=0.64$). The author concludes from the results that the indication for adenotomy must be individual and, depending on the severity of the complaints and possible complications, can be delayed for several months because spontaneous resolutions are possible (EBM evidence grade 1b).

▪ Bronchial Asthma and Allergic Asthma

Bronchial asthma is the chronic condition that is most frequently diagnosed in GP practices. In Germany, 10% of children and ca. 5% of adults suffer from it (ZKV[4] 1998). Various pathophysiological mechanisms that can be divided into immunological and non-immunological

---

4   ZKV – Zentralinstitut für kassenärztliche Versorgung (Central institute for insurance-covered healthcare in Germany)

stimuli – although a mixture of both can be present – are responsible for an inflammation of the respiratory tract leading to recurring episodes of dyspnoea, chest tightness and cough with wheezing, especially in the night and early in the morning.

Diagnosis is based on clinical information about frequency and severity of attacks as well as on apparative examination (such as peak-flow measurement, spirometry test, etc.).

Therapy plans depend on genesis and stage of asthma (cf. treatment guidelines of the German Medical Association's Drug Commission; AVP[5] 1st edn 2001). The WHO categorisation differentiates four stages: stage 1 with up to two daytime symptoms per week and less than two nocturnal symptoms per month with normal pulmonary function. A corresponding increase in the frequency of attacks with normal pulmonary function at rest defines stages 2 and 3. In stage 4 complaints are persistent due to constant and often severe exacerbations, with pulmonary function being restricted to an extent that activities have to be limited (Bassler et al. 1998). In terms of treatment there is medication on demand and permanent medication. Medicinal treatment essentially includes bronchodilators (especially β2-sympathomimetic agents with long- or short-term effects as well as theophyllines, anticholinergic and antileukotriene agents) and glucocorticoids.

▪▪ Studies:

25. Lewith et al. (2002). Use of ultramolecular potencies of allergen to treat asthmatic people allergic to house dust mite: double-blind randomized controlled clinical trial

The trial examined the effectiveness of homeopathic immunotherapy against placebo in 242 asthma patients. The results show a significant advantage for the homeopathic treatment for three of seven parameters, i.e. the severity of asthma symptoms (assessed via VAS, $p=0.047$), mood ($p=0.013$) and matutinal peak expiratory flow ($p=0.025$). The authors nevertheless consider the differences to be clinically insignificant and conclude that homeopathic treatment of allergic asthma is not effective (EBM evidence grade 1b).

26. Eizayaga and Eizayaga (1996). Homeopathic treatment of bronchial asthma

The retrospective study examined the effects of individualized homeopathic treatment over a minimum of 8 months with 62 asthma patients. Comparison before and after treatment showed significant improvement in the severity of the disease and frequency of attacks. Before treatment, 64.5% of patients had at least one attack per month and 35.5% between two and 11 attacks per year, with 90.3% of them reporting moderate to severe attacks. After treatment, 25.8% of patients had no attacks, a further 25.8% had up to one attack per year and 22.6% had two to 11 attacks per year with the severity of attacks being described as 'mild' by 56.5% and as 'moderate to severe' by 17.7% of the patients. Only 11.3% of patients reported no improvement after treatment. In addition, the termination of conventional medication was documented: corticosteroids with 13/18 patients (corresponding to 72.2%), theophylline with 10/14 (71.4%) and β2-adrenergic agents with 9/31 (29%). Despite the methodical limitations of a retrospective assessment, the results reflect the effectiveness of the treatment experienced daily by homeopaths and support the demand for further research. They also emphasize the importance of selecting the right medicine, as effectiveness could otherwise be restricted (EBM evidence grade 3).

---

5   AVP – Arzneiverordnung in der Praxis (Pharmaceutical prescriptions in the medical practice)

27. Matusiewicz and Rotkiewicz-Piorun (1997). Behandlung schwerer Formen von kortikoid-abhängigem Bronchialasthma mit Immunsuppressiva und antihomotoxischen Mitteln
The controlled clinical study examined the treatment of 50 children with corticoid-dependent asthma with immunosuppressives in combination with Traumeel S® and Engystol® N or placebo. The results suggest that corticoid medication could be significantly reduced in the homeopathically treated group compared with the placebo group. The whole study structure was very unclear, however; it appears that before-after comparisons were carried out. No clear differences were shown for laboratory parameters (EBM evidence grade 2a).

28. Reilly et al. (1994). Is evidence for homeopathy reproducible?
To reproduce the evidence from two previous trials, 28 patients with allergic asthma were treated with homeopathy or placebo (in addition to their usual conventional treatment) in a randomized controlled trial. A daily overall symptom score showed an advantage for the homeopathically treated group within a week of treatment begin (p=0.003). Measurements of respiratory function and bronchial reactivity were the same for both groups. A meta-analysis of this and the two previous trials showed a significant positive effect for the homeopathic treatment (p=0.0004) (EBM evidence grade 1a/b).

29. White et al. (2003) Individualized homeopathy as an adjunct in the treatment of childhood asthma: a randomized placebo controlled trial
In this double-blind trial the effects of individualized homeopathic treatment were examined in 96 children with asthma as an adjunct to their conventional therapy. Success was measured in terms of quality of life after 12 months, based on the childhood asthma questionnaire, and showed no difference between the groups. For other parameters such as the use of inhalation devices and days off school there was no difference between the groups either. In the homeopathically treated group 13 adverse events occurred in 12 children, and in the placebo group ten adverse events in ten children, one of which led to withdrawal from the trial. The paper does not include a categorisation of medication. The reported symptoms suggest the possibility of initial aggravations in the homeopathically treated group. The authors conclude that the trial does not provide evidence that individualized homeopathic treatment as an adjunct improves the quality of life in childhood asthma (EBM evidence grade 1b).

10.3 Summary of Studies: Data Extraction, Internal and External Validity, Results

10.3.1 Population, study design and implementation

The various indications are spread as follows among the 29 trials that were evaluated: otitis media (6 trials), allergic rhinitis (5), influenza-like infections (4), bronchial asthma (4), URTI/A (3), sinusitis (2), adenoid vegetations (1), infectious mononucleosis (1), cough (1), allergic asthma (1) and tonsillitis (1).

Of the 23 controlled trials, 17 were randomized. For ten of these the method of randomisation is considered 'adequate', for another two trials 'possibly adequate' and for five trials randomisation was 'not documented'. Six studies were controlled but not randomized, five were cohort studies and one was a single case report (cf. ◘ Fig. 10.2).

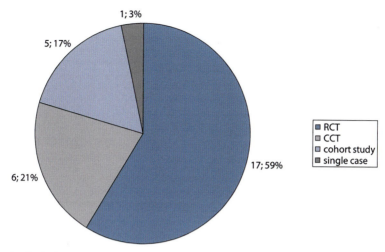

Fig. 10.2 Study design. Number and frequency (*n*; %) of trials

Of the 23 controlled trials, 14 were compared with placebo; in nine trials the control group received conventional treatment. Fifteen trials were blinded, with 14 being double-blind (physician and patient) and one single-blind (patient). The number of treatment groups per study ranged from 'one group' (five trials), through 'two groups' (20 trials) and 'three groups' (two trials) to 'four groups' (one trial); one publication was a single case description.

Of the controlled trials ten had 'comparable' treatment groups at trial begin; for nine studies they were only 'possibly comparable' and for two 'not comparable'. In two cases the documentation was not sufficient to establish comparability.

Documentation of 'dropouts' and 'lost to follow-up' is adequate in ten trials, 'possibly adequate' in five and 'not adequate' in another five trials. For seven trials there was no information in this respect. Two trials (one retrospective and one single case) could not be evaluated in this category.

For two of the trials that show only a trend for the homeopathic group compared with the control group reservations apply due to low case numbers. The authors confirm that the case number calculated was too low (Weber et al. 2002 and Jacobs et al. 2001).

10.3.2 **Intervention and control therapy**

Information on the homeopathic method applied was divided into four categories: classical, individualized treatment (11), clinical homeopathy (4), complex homeopathy (7) and isopathy (7) (cf. **Fig. 10.3**). The validity of symptoms was taken into account in six trials; in 24 trials it was not considered or not documented.

The similarity principle was applied in nine trials, in four trials only partly, in 16 trials either not at all or it was not documented.

Confounding factors for the homeopathic treatment were definitely considered in two trials, in two further trials it was 'possibly considered'. Based on the treatment protocols, seven trials

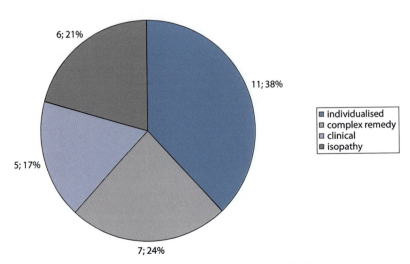

■ **Fig. 10.3** Homeopathic treatment categories. Number and frequency (n; %) of trials

appear not to have considered confounding factors. With 18 trials there was no documentation on this account.

Of the 23 controlled trials, 14 were compared with placebo and nine with conventional treatment. One trial compared its own results with those published by a placebo-controlled trial (Frei et al. 2001).

10.3.3 Outcome

Outcome parameters were said to be 'predefined' in 27 trials. For ten trials the primary parameter was described as purely 'clinical', in five trials clinical parameters were assessed in connection with quality of life and in three trials in connection with 'costs'. Eight trials assessed surrogate parameters + clinical parameters, one study assessed only surrogate parameters and one only quality of life. One study included surrogate + clinical parameters + quality of life in its outcome evaluation (cf. ■ Fig. 10.4).

10.3.4 Results

The observational studies and the single case report showed positive results for homeopathy. When compared with conventional treatment, six of seven trials proved to be equivalent, in only one trial (penicillin treatment for streptococcal tonsillitis vs. homeopathy) was homeopathy inferior. Eight of the 16 placebo-controlled studies, , i.e. 50%, showed a significant result in favour of homeopathy, though none of them used individualized treatment; four trials showed a trend and four no advantage. All in all, 24 of 29 trials were positive and showed significance or a trend in favour of homeopathy in the course of treatment when compared with placebo, or significance, a trend or equivalence when compared with conventional standard treatment (cf. ■ Tables 10.1–10.4).

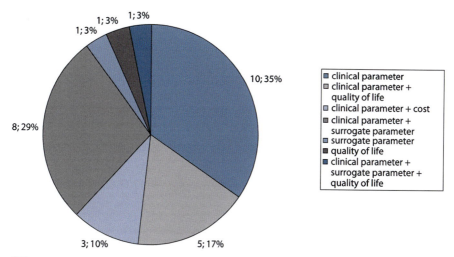

Fig. 10.4 Categories of outcome parameters: number and frequency (n; %) of trials

Legend:
- clinical parameter
- clinical parameter + quality of life
- clinical parameter + cost
- clinical parameter + surrogate parameter
- surrogate parameter
- quality of life
- clinical parameter + surrogate parameter + quality of life

Comments on the clinical trials including an evaluation of the external validity (EV) are also charted in ▫ Tables 10.1–10.3. ▫ Table 10.4 contains a detailed EV evaluation.

Only four trials showed good external validity, one of them being a study of individualized treatment with significant superiority over conventional treatment. One clinical homeopathy study and one complex homeopathy study showed significance compared with placebo. The fourth study was a single case description.

10.3.5 Side effects, initial aggravation, adverse effects

Documentation of side effects was considered 'adequate' in 13 trials, 'possibly adequate' in four and 'not adequate' in three; nine trials did not mention side effects.

For the evaluation of results and side effects, homeopathic criteria were considered in only three trials; with 26 trials nothing was documented in this respect.

If initial aggravation, a well-known phenomenon in classical homeopathy, occurs, the symptoms arising can be seen as indicating effectiveness of the homeopathic treatment. Initial aggravation was documented by Taylor et al. (2000).

The study by Herzberger et al. (1997) documents, in addition to the low incidence of side effects, the compatibility of homeopathic and conventional treatment.

10.4 Discussion

Overall evaluation: documentation, internal and external validity:
Evaluation of 29 trials on the indication upper respiratory tract infection/allergic reactions (URTI/A) that included clinical studies of various designs showed an overall positive result in 24 of the 29. The positive trend persisted when particular subgroups were evaluated. If only the placebo-controlled, randomized trials with the highest EBM evidence are considered, 12 of 16

trials show a positive result for the homeopathically treated group (significantly positive 8/16 and trend 4/16). When compared with conventional treatment, 6/7 trials show a positive result (significantly positive 1/7 and equivalence with conventional treatment 5/7). Overall, the reviewers rated the quality of documentation 'good' for 13 trials, 'medium' for ten and 'poor' for six.

If documentation was poor, internal and external validity were not evaluable, which means that only 23 trials could be assessed for their validity: internal validity was rated 'good' in ten trials, 'medium' in ten and 'poor' in three. External validity was considered 'good' in six trials, 'medium' in 12 and 'poor' in five.

If one takes into account the reduced external validity of the randomized trials due to selection of participants and blinding, both of which impair the effectiveness of classical homeopathy, the trial results still clearly indicate clinical efficacy of homeopathy. The positive effect is apparent not only in the placebo-controlled trials but also in comparison to conventional therapies.

For the ten trials that applied the classical homeopathic concept of individualized treatment the following picture emerges:

The two randomized, placebo-controlled trials showed a trend for the homeopathic treatment. Of the two randomized trials that compared classical homeopathic treatment with conventional medicine, one showed a 'trend for homeopathic therapy' and the other 'no difference' between the two treatment groups.

Some trials investigated the use of conventional medication as a secondary outcome parameter next to clinical symptoms and findings from instrument tests. Friese et al. (1997c) and Frei (2001) both registered a definite decrease in antibiotic consumption for the homeopathically treated groups. The trial by Eizayaga and Eizayaga (1996) showed that homeopathic treatment as an adjunct for corticosteroid-dependent asthma resulted in a reduction of conventional medication and alleviation of the obviously severe side effects caused by conventional medicines. Similar results were reported by Matusiewicz and Rotkiewicz-Piorin (1997). These results are significant not only clinically (e.g. by supporting the demand for a more **targeted** use of antibiotics in the face of increasing resistance) but also economically, as the homeopathic medication used is much more cost-effective.

With regard to the transferability of trial results, the external validity – which depends on the particular context of the HTA, in this case the situation in Switzerland – needs to be taken into account. The following bias factors and restrictions to the transferability of study results to everyday medical practice as it exists in Switzerland might apply in this case:

- Selection of patients for participation in randomized trials
- Blinding can cause insecurity with regard to the therapeutic context and lead to loss of trust, which can diminish effectiveness.
- Physicians taking part in the trial might not be adequately trained in homeopathy to be able to choose and implement effective homeopathic treatment. This applies in particular to classical homeopathy, where even the diagnosis follows a specialized procedure that is necessary for identification of the effective remedy.
- Case numbers are too small.
- Assessment of 'subjective' symptoms in unblinded trials

Transferability of the results of a randomized study design is generally restricted due to the high selection of patients and the blinding of physician and patient (see Chap. 5). The experimental study structure can cause the kind of effect impairment that is usually observed in the clinical situation. Other possible negative influences are described in Chap. 9. Despite these restrictions probable effectiveness can be concluded from the study results available.

Eizayaga and Eizayaga (1996) also mention the question of the adequacy of the trial physicians' homeopathic training and experience and request that homeopathic treatment be carried out exclusively by trained and experienced physicians, as effectiveness might otherwise be reduced due to incorrect substance selection.

The trials that were examined focus on epidemiologically and economically significant disorders, some of which find little consideration in conventional medical research. The request for a stronger presence of general practitioners in research that Wiesenauer et al. (1989) put forward has therefore not lost any of its relevance. They point out that the general practitioners with their knowledge about practice-relevant diseases and about the effectiveness of available treatments are often not considered in clinical trials.

Conclusion:
In the trials that were examined, the internal as well as external validity and thus the transferability of results to the situation in Switzerland were restricted due to various factors which do not, however, put the effectiveness of homeopathic treatment in general in doubt. Notwithstanding the study design, the trial results showed probable effectiveness of homeopathy for allergies and infectious diseases of the upper respiratory tract. Tolerability of the treatment is very good and is not reduced through combination with conventional treatment. Economic advantages are possible due to the fact that homeopathic treatment can lessen the need for conventional medication. The trials reveal further implications for practice-related research. The 29 evaluated trials show mostly positive evidence of effectiveness for homeopathy. As mentioned at the beginning, identification and retrieval of literature is very problematic, and we later heard of other articles which would have satisfied the inclusion criteria but which we did not detect at the time despite our elaborate search strategy. Our search was also not extended to include countries such as India, where the use of homeopathy is widespread. It can therefore be assumed that a more comprehensive investigation would further increase the amount of positive evidence.

■ **Table 10.1** Primary studies with homeopathic intervention for indication upper respiratory tract infections/allergic reactions (URTI/A) without control

Authors, year	Study type	No. of cases	Homeopathic intervention	Indication
Bahemann 2002	single case	1	individualized: Kalium chromatum C 200	pharyngitis, tonsillitis, inf. mononucleosis
Eizayaga and Eizayaga 1996	application (observational) (retrospective)	62	individualized	bronchial asthma, allergic asthma
Frei and Thurneysen 2001	application (observational)	230	individualized	acute otitis media (AOM)
Friese 1994	application (observational	30	individualized	otitis media
Herzberger and Weiser 1997	application (observational	1 479	complex: Engystol N®	URTI general
Rabe 2001	application (observational	339	complex: Husteel®	cough

n.e.: not evaluable, EV external validity

■ **Table 10.2** Primary studies with homeopathic intervention for indication upper respiratory tract infections/allergic reactions (URTI/A) with conventional medical control

Authors, year	Study type	No. of cases	Homeopathic intervention/ conventional intervention	Indication
Friese et al (1997c)	CCT	131	individualized vs. nasal drops, secretolytics, antipyretics (also individualized)	otitis media
Gassinger et al. 1981	RCT	53	clinical, Eupatorium perfoliatum D2 vs. Aspirin	flu-like infection
Harrison et al. 1999	RCT	33	homeopathic vs. conventional treatment (no further information)	otitis media with hearing loss and effusion
Maiwald et al. 1998 ▼	RCT	170	complex, Gripp-Heel® vs. ASS (acetylsalicylic acid)	influenza-like infection

10

Result (response rate)	EBM-grade	EV	Comments
treatment successful	4	+	Documentation good; local symptom description only
64.5% (before-after-treatment difference $p<0.001$)	3	+/-	Classical homeopathy; good general description, but description of population deficient.
72% in total; 39% after 6 h and 33% after 12 h	3	+/-	The trial was conducted at a time when all children with AOM received antibiotic treatment. The homeopathy criteria for external validity were fully observed. The possible influence of the adjunct analgesic medication after 6 h is not discussed. From information published on placebo control a 2.4 times higher success rate was calculated for the homeopathic treatment. No reference is made to the comparability of study populations and to the selection criteria for comparative studies. Treatment costs as a secondary parameter reveal the potential for savings.
73%	3	n.e.	Single remedy, but application extremely schematized. Interesting as pilot study, usability of results restricted. Effectiveness likely according to clinical results; 17/30 lost to follow-up, of which only 3/30 are not seen as successful.
50–90% (depending on symptoms)	3	n.e.	Documentation deficient, also for criteria relevant to homeopathy.
95%	3	n.e.	Heterogeneous population; many adjunct therapies impede evaluation.

Result	EBM grade	EV	Comments
equivalent or trend for homeopathy	2a	+/-	Different group sizes lower evaluability of results (103 homeopathy, 28 conventional medicine).
equivalent	1b	n.e.	Study was not blinded.
equivalent or trend for homeopathy	1b	+/-	Patient group too small; high risk of performance and detection bias; problem of unblinded randomisation.
equivalent or trend for homeopathy	1b	-	Risk of bias relatively high (possible un-blinding, estimated ASS success rate not achieved, selection criteria not uniform, result therefore difficult to assess. No p-values given.

□ Table 10.2 (continued)

Authors, year	Study type	No. of cases	Homeopathic intervention/ conventional intervention	Indication
Nusche 1998	CCT	51	individualized vs. penicillin	pharyngitis, tonsillitis with streptococcal infection
Riley et al. 2001	CCT	456	individualized vs. conventional treatment (no further information given)	URTI general
Weber et al. 2002	CCT	63	Clinical with possibility of individualized treatment (mostly Cinnabaris D3 + Sinupret) vs. antibiotics, secretolytics, xylometazoline (individual decision)	sinusitis

n.e.: not evaluable; CCT: controlled clinical trial; RCT: randomized clinical trial; IV: internal validity; EV: external validit

□ Table 10.3 Primary studies with homeopathic intervention for indication upper respiratory tract infections/ allergic reactions (URTI/A) with placebo control

Authors, year	Study type	No. of cases	Homeopathic intervention	Indication
Aabel 2000	RCT	80	isopathy (Betula C30)	rhinitis (allergy to birch pollen)
de Lange de Klerk et al. 1994	RCT	175	individualized	URTI general
Ferley et al. 1989	RCT	478	clinical (Oscillococcinum, no detailed information)	influenza-like infection
Friese et al. 2001	RCT	97	clinical (four single remedies in succession)	adenoid vegetation
Jacobs et al. 2001a ▼	RCT	75	individualized	otitis media

Result	EBM grade	EV	Comments
no advantage, significance for penicillin	2a	n.e.	Overall documentation is poor so that neither IV nor EV can be reliably evaluated; basically no information on evaluation. Due to information regarding the homeopathic training of the physicians it can be assumed that the study had good model validity.
significance for homeopathy	2b	+	
equivalent or trend for homeopathy	2a	+/-	Adjunct medication might confound homeopathy group. No adjustment made although groups were different.

Result	EBM grade	EV	Comments
no advantage	1b	-	Diagnosis not established according to HP criteria, confounding factors not always observed; uncommon form of treatment (prevention); strong selection of patients, as co-morbidity reason for exclusion; adjunct medication permitted: topical and systemic antihistamines; low pollen count in study year (colder and wetter than usual) might have prevented or reduced symptoms compared with other years. Comparability of groups restricted at baseline (previous unconventional treatment: in the homeopathy group 14, in the control group only six patients), no information as to whether this was considered in analysis.
trend for homeopathy	1b	+	Good study design, adequate method for homeopathy but no details on homeopathic treatment; not enough patients to prove effectiveness (lack of power).
significance for homeopathy	1b	+/-	Patients from 149 general practices in the Rhône-Alpes region, France, with influenza-like symptoms, mixed practices, mostly not homeopathic
no advantage (high placebo response rates)	1b	+/-	Groups not comparable in terms of disease parameters. No adjustment mentioned for evaluation. No dropouts. In the placebo group the surgery indication was not upheld either: 63.8% (homeopathy group 66%)
trend for primary, significance for secondary parameter	1b	+/-	Author refers to relatively low case number, which could be responsible for trend only.

Table 10.3 (continued)

Authors, year	Study type	No. of cases	Homeopathic intervention	Indication
Lewith et al. 2002	RCT	242	isopathy (potentized house dust mites)	allergic asthma
Matusiewicz and Rotkiewicz-Piorun 1997	CCT	50 (6-arm!)	complex (Engystol N® + Traumeel®), in addition to immunosuppressants cyclosporin A, methotrexate, analogue as control; placebo in various combinations	corticoid-dependent allergic asthma
Mössinger 1985	CCT	44 (38 evaluated)	clinical (Pulsatilla D2)	otitis media, secretory otitis media
Papp and Schuback 1998	RCT	372	clinical; Oscillococcinum without further information	influenza-like infections
Reilly and Taylor 1985	RCT	39	isopathy (grass pollen C30)	allergic rhinitis
Reilly et al. 1986	RCT	158 (144 treated)	isopathy (grass pollen C30)	allergic rhinitis
Reilly et al. 1994	RCT	28	isopathy (of the individual allergen)	allergic asthma
Taylor et al. 2000	RCT	51	isopathy (C30 preparation of specific allergen)	allergic rhinitis
White et al. 2003	RCT	36	individualized, adjunct to conventional treatment vs. placebo + conventional treatment	childhood asthma
Wiesenauer and Gaus 1985	RCT	164 (3-arm)	clinical (Galphimia D6)	allergic rhinitis
Wiesenauer et al. 1989	RCT	152 (4-arm)	complex (Luffa operculta D4, Kalium bichromatum D4, Cinnabaris D3, partly in combination)	sinusitis

n.e.: not evaluable; CCT: controlled clinical trial; RCT: randomized clinical trial; EV external validity

Result	EBM grade	EV	Comments
significance for homeopathy (but differences not clinically relevant)	1b	+	Study planning very precise.
significance for homeopathy (but before-after-treatment difference for 21 outcome parameters)	2a	-	Information on randomisation, blinding, group composition etc. not sufficient for evaluation!, case number very low at 5–11 patients per treatment arm, study structure unclear
significance for homeopathy	1b	n.e.	Diagnostics unclear; homeopathic training of physicians not clear; homeopathy diagnostics unclear. Altogether little information given.
significance for homeopathy	1b	+/-	Meticulous analysis with no apparent detection bias.
trend for homeopathy	1b	+/-	Paper mentions that the treating physicians were trained homeopaths with at least 5 years of practical experience; group size too small, randomisation and blinding weak; study meaningful, as it was used as a basis for further studies!
significance for homeopathy	1b	+/-	Participating physicians used homeopathy on average in 18% of cases, nine physicians in less than 10% and three physicians so far no homeopathy. Documentation of results is relatively precise, although it is not clear how the loss to follow-up is included in the analysis.
significance for homeopathy	1b	+/-	Not all participating physicians were homeopaths. Study implementation was good, apart from too small patient numbers. Selection of patients after randomisation for further trial participation not clearly described. A meta-analysis was conducted on the results of this and two earlier trials, which also showed a significantly positive result for homeopathy.
significance for homeopathy	1b	+/-	Initial aggravation was observed frequently for homeopathy group, which is seen as indicating effectiveness of the homeopathic treatment, not as a side effect!
no advantage	1b	+/-	Positive tendency noticeable with more severe asthma. For some secondary parameters evaluation revealed 'trend for the treatment', but number of cases too low to allow for further conclusions.
trend for homeopathy	1b	+/-	Quality and precision of description deficient: baseline data in some cases mention fewer patients than the outcome tables! No explanation given.
no advantage	1b	-	Loss rate is very high at 31% (main reasons: wrongly filled in questionnaires and medication that was not permitted). The latter constitutes breach of protocol and should be further analysed. Due to subgroup evaluation (acute and chronic sinusitis) case numbers are too small to allow for a reliable conclusion.

10

▫ Table 10.4 Information on aspects of homeopathic treatment in selected studies on the domain URTI

Authors, year	Basic study population	Homeopathic treatment	Weight of symptoms documented	Similarity rule observed	Con-founding factors observed
Aabel 2000	recruitment via news-paper adverts (Oslo)	isopathy	no	no	yes
Bahemann 2002	(single case)	individualized	n.d.	yes	no
de Lange de Klerk et al. 1994	homeopathic care in university outpatient clinic, conventional care by conventional physician (recruitment: general practitioner + press)	individualized	yes	yes	partly
Eizayaga & Eizayaga 1996	62 cases from homeo-pathically treated patients of the Fundación HOMEOS Institute in Buenos Aires	individualized	yes	yes	n.d.
Ferley et al. 1989	patients from various practices, mostly not homeopathic physicians	isopathy	no	no	partly
Frei 2001	children and adolescents from a practice with specialized homeopathy	individualized	yes	yes	yes
Friese 1994	patients of an ENT practice, mostly homeo-pathically treated	individualized	yes	partly	no
Friese et al.1997c)	children from ENT and paediatric practices, one homeopathy practice and four conventional ENT practices from the Stuttgart area/ Germany	individualized	no	yes	n.d.
Friese et al. 2001	patients referred to the Friese ENT practice in Weil der Stadt/ Germany	complex remedy	n.d.	partly	n.d.
Gassinger et al. 1981	patients of a general practice in Germany	clinical	no	no	n.d.
Harrison et al. 1999 ▼	n.d.	individualized	no	yes	n.d.

◘ Table 10.4 (continued)

Authors, year	Basic study population	Homeopathic treatment	Weight of symptoms documented	Similarity rule observed	Con-founding factors observed
Herzberger and Weiser 1997	154 physicians in private practice (136 GPs, nine paediatricians, eight ENT, one surgeon) from three countries	complex remedy	no	n.d.	no
Jacobs et al. 2001	private group of children, paediatrician practice (Seattle, WA)	individualized	n.d.	yes	n.d.
Lewith et al. 2002	patients from 38 GP practices (South-hampton)	isopathy	no	no	no
Maiwald et al. 1988	German army regular soldiers and conscripts aged 17–49, with influenza-like infection on sick leave	complex remedy	no	no	n.d.
Matusiewicz and Rotkiewicz-Piorun 1997	asthma patients from a hospital	complex remedy	n.d.	n.d.	n.d.
Mössinger 1985	patients from seven paediatric and six general practices (private)	clinical	n.d.	n.d.	n.d.
Nusche 1998	All patients aged 3–14 were invited to participate. No detailed documentation of the setting given.	individualized	n.d.	n.d.	n.d.
Papp and Schulback 1998	15–20 general medical and internist practices in Germany	isopathy	no	no	no
Rabe 2001	Patients from 71 practices (general medical and paediatric)	complex remedy	no	no	no
Reilly et al. 1994	out-patient clinic (West Central Scotland)	isopathy	no	partly	n.d.
Reilly and Taylor 1985 ▼	15 NHS GP practices	isopathy	n.d.	n.d.	n.d.

□ Table 10.4 (continued)

Authors, year	Basic study population	Homeopathic treatment	Weight of symptoms documented	Similarity rule observed	Con-founding factors observed
Reilly et al. 1986	two homeopathic hospitals in Glasgow and London, 26 NHS GPs, recruited 1984	clinical	no	no	n.d.
Riley et al. 2001	primary care centres from four countries, six hospitals, all patients with three symptom pictures	individualized	yes	yes	n.d.
Taylor et al. 2000	four ENT practices and ENT outpatient clinic of Northwick Park Hospital	isopathy	n.d.	n.d.	n.d.
Weber et al. 2002	five ENT practices, three conventional, two CAM specialists' practices in a city with pre-selected patient populations	complex remedy	n.d.	no	n.d.
White et al. 2003	five practices in Somerset (UK)	individualized	no	yes	no
Wiesenauer and Gaus 1985	75 German (mostly general medical practices	clinical	no	no	n.d.
Wiesenauer et al. 1989	47 private practices (general medical and internist) in West Germany with and without complementary homeopathy	complex	No	partly	n.d.

CAM: complementary alternative medicine; GP: general practitioner; n.d.: not documented

10

▣ **Table 10.5** Domain URTI/A: excluded studies plus reason

First author, year	Title	Reason for exclusion
Asher 2001	Complementary and alternative medicine in otolaryngology	Systematic review
Barnett 2000	Challenges of evaluating homeopathic treatment of acute otitis media	The study's objective is to improve the study design, not to examine the efficacy of homeopathic therapies.
Dunn 1997	Homeopathic-alternative medication (HAM) in the treatment of seasonal allergic rhinitis	Abstract only, documentation is not sufficient for evaluation
Frenkel 2002	Effects of homeopathic intervention on medication consumption in atopic and allergic disorders	Indication is much wider than URTI. Study examined whether use of conventional medication decreased after homeopathic treatment and if costs were reduced.
Friese et al. 1996	Acute otitis media in children. Comparison between conventional and homeopathic therapy	Double publication with Friese 1997c 'The homeopathic treatment of acute otitis media in children – comparison with conventional therapy'
Friese 1997	Quality assurance in homeopathy shown on the example of adenoid vegetations	Double publication with 1. Friese et al. 'Homeopathic treatment of adenoid vegetations. Results of a prospective, randomized...' (1997b); Journal 'HNO' 2. Friese et al. 'Results of a randomized prospective double-blind clinical trial…" (2001)
Friese et al. 1997b	Homeopathic treatment of adenoid vegetations. Result of a prospective, randomized double-blind study	Double publication
Rabe 2001	Treatment of cough of different genesis with a modern homeopathic preparation	The study examines not the efficacy of homeopathic therapy but the reasons for using homeopathy.

10.5   References

Aabel S (2000) No beneficial effect of isopathic prophylactic treatment for birch pollen allergy during a low-pollen season: a double-blind placebo-controlled clinical trial of homeopathic Betula 30c. Br Homeopathic J 89:169–173

Agency for Health Care Policy and Research (AHCPR) (1992) Acute pain management: operative and medical procedures and trauma. Clinical practice guideline no 1. AHCPR Publication No. 92-0023, Appendix B. available at: http://www.ncbi.nlm.nih.gov/books/bv.fcgi?rid=hstat6.table.9286

Asher BFM, Seidman MM, Snyderman CM (2001) Complementary and alternative medicine in otolaryngology. Laryngoscope 111:1383–1389

Bahemann A (2002) Kalium bromatum bei infektioser Mononukleose. Z Klassische Homöopathie 46:232–233

Barnett ED, Levatin JL, Chapman EH, Floyd LA, Eisenberg D, Kaptchuk TJ et al (2000) Challenges of evaluating homeopathic treatment of acute otitis media. Pediatr Infect Dis J 19:273–275

Bassler D, Antes G, Forster J (1998)Leitlinienbericht "Asthma bronchiale". Ärztliche Zentralstelle für Qualitätssicherung

Burke P, Bain J, Robinson D, Dunn JM (1991) Acute red ear in children: controlled trial of non-antibiotic treatment in general practice. BMJ 303:558–562

De Lange de Klerk ESM, Blommers J, Kruik DJ, Bezemer PD, Feenstra L (1994) Effect of homeopathic medicines on daily burden of symptoms in children with recurrent upper respiratory tract infections. BMJ 309:1329–1332

Dunn JM, DeMasi JM (1997) Homeopathic-alternative medication (HAM) in the treatment of seasonal allergic rhinitis (SAR). J Allergy Clin Immunol 99:61

Eizayaga FX, Eizayaga J (1996) Homeopathic treatment of bronchial asthma. Retrospective study of 62 cases. Br Homeopathic J 85:28–33

Ferley JP, Zmirou D, D'Adhemar D, Balducci F (1989) A controlled evaluation of a homeopathic preparation in the treatment of influenza-like syndromes. Br J Clin Pharmacol 27:329–336

Frei H, Thurneysen A (2001) Homeopathy in acute otitis media in children: treatment effect or spontaneous resolution? Br Homeopathic J 90:180–182

Frenkel M HD (2002) Effects of homeopathic intervention on medication consumption in atopic and allergic disorders. Altern Ther Health Med 8:76–79

Friese KH (1994) The homeopathic therapy of acute otitis media in children [in German]. Therapiewoche 44:348–353

Friese KH (1997) Qualitätssicherung in der Homöopathie am Beispiel der adenoiden Vegetationen. Allgemeine Homöopathische Zeitung 242:68–72

Friese KH, Kruse S, Moeller H (1996) Otitis media in children. A comparison of conventional and homeopathic drugs [in German]. HNO 44:462–466

Friese KH, Kruse S, Moeller H (1997a) Acute otitis media in children: a comparison of conventional and homeopathic treatment. Biomed Ther 15:113–116

Friese KH, Feuchter U, Moeller H (1997b) Homeopathic treatment of adenoid vegetations. Results of a prospective, randomized double-blind study. HNO 45:618–624

Friese KH, Kruse S, Lüdtke R, Moeller H (1997c) The homeopathic treatment of otitis media in children – Comparisons with conventional therapy. International J Clin Pharmacol Therapeutics 35:296–301

Friese KH, Feuchter U, Lüdtke R, Moeller H (2001) Results of a randomized prospective double-blind clinical trial on the homeopathic treatment of adenoid vegetations. Eur J General Practice 7:48–54

Gassinger CA, Wunstel G, Netter P (1981) A controlled clinical trial for testing the efficacy of the homeopathic drug eupatorium perfoliatum D2 in the treatment of common cold. [German]. Arzneimittelforschung 31:732–736

Haidvogl M (1993) Klinische Studien zum Wirksamkeitsnachweis der Homöopathie. Dtsch Apothekerzeitung 133:1697–1705

Harrison H., Fixsen A, Vickers A (1999) A randomized comparison of homeopathic and standard care for the treatment of glue ear in children. Complement Ther Med 7:132–135

Herzberger G, Weiser M (1997) Homeopathic treatment of infections of various origins: a prospective study. Biomed Ther 15:123–127

Jacobs J, Springer DA, Crothers D (2001) Homeopathic treatment of acute otitis media in children: A preliminary randomized placebo-controlled trial. Pediatr Infect Dis J 20:177–183

Kruse S (2004) Otitis media bei Kindern – Homöopathie versus konventionelle Therapie. Hippokrates Verlag, Stuttgart

Lewith GT, Watkins AD, Hyland ME, Shaw S, Broomfield JA, Dolan G, Holgate ST (2002) Use of ultramolecular potencies of allergen to treat asthmatic people allergic to house dust mite: double blind randomized controlled clinical trial. BMJ 324:520–523. doi:10.1136/bmj.324.7336.520

Linde K, Clausius N, Ramirez G, Melchart D, Eitel F, Hedges LV, et al (1997) Are the clinical effects of homeopathy placebo effects? A meta-analysis of placebo-controlled trials. Lancet 350:834–843

Linde K, Melchart D (1998) Randomized controlled trials of individualized homeopathy: a state-of-the-art review. J Altern Complement Med 4:371–388

Maiwald L, Weinfurtner T, Mau J, Connert WD (1988) Treatment of common cold with a combination homeopathic preparation compared with acetylsalicylic acid. Controlled randomized single-blind study. Arzneimittelforschung 38:578–582

Matusiewicz R, Rokiewicz-Piorun A (1997) Behandlung schwerer Formen von kortikoidabhängigem Bronchialasthma mit Immunsuppressiva und antihomotoxischen Mitteln. Biol Med 26:67–72

Mössinger P (1985) Zur Behandlung der Otitis media mit Pulsatilla. Kinderarzt 16:581–582

Nusche M (1998) Homöopathie oder Penicilin bei Mandelentzündungen? Eine prospektive klinische Studie. Hippokrates Verlag, Stuttgart

Ollenschläger G, Helou A, Lorenz W (2000) Kritische Bewertung von Leitlinien. In: Kunz R, Ollenschläger G, Raspe HH (eds) Lehrbuch evidenzbasierte Medizin in Klinik und Praxis. Schriftenreihe Hans Neuffer Stiftung, Deutscher ÄrzteVerlag, Köln, pp 156-176

Papp R, Schuback G (1998) Oscillococcinum® in patients with influenza-like syndroms: a placebo-controlled double-blind evaluation. Br Homeopathic J 87:69–76

Rabe A (2001) Treatment of cough of different genesis with a modern homeopathic preparation. [in German]. Biol Med 30:234–238

Reilly D, Taylor MA, Beattie NG, Campbell JH, McSharry C, Aitchison TC, Carter R, Stevenson R (1994) Is evidence for homeopathy reproducible? Lancet 344:1601–1606

Reilly DT, McSharry C, Taylor MA, Aitchison T (1986) Is homeopathy a placebo response? Controlled trial of homeopathic potency with pollen in hay fever as model. Lancet 2:881–886

Reilly DT, Taylor MA (1985) Potent placebo or potency? A proposed study model with initial findings using homeopathically prepared pollens in hayfever. Br Homeopathic J 74:65–74

Righetti M (1988) Forschung in der Homöopathie. Grundlagen, Problematik und Ergebnisse. Burgdorf, Göttingen

Riley D, Fischer M, Singh B, Haidvogl M, Heger M (2001) Homeopathy and conventional medicine: an outcomes study comparing effectiveness in a primary care setting. J Altern Complement Med 7:149–159

SIGN 50 (Scottish Intercollegiate Guidelines Network) (2004) A guideline developers' handbook (Sect. 6). Edinburgh available at: http://www.sign.ac.uk/guidelines/fulltext/50/section6.html

Smyrnios NA, Irwin RS, Curley FJ, French CL (1998) From a prospective study of chronic cough. Arch Intern Med 158:1222–1228

Taylor MA, Reilly D, Llewellyn-Jones RH, McSharry C, Aitchison TC (2000) Randomized controlled trial of homeopathy versus placebo in perennial allergic rhinitis with overview of four trial series. BMJ 21:471–476

Walach H, Righetti M (1996) Homeopathy – foundations, research and strategies of evaluation. Wien Klin Wochenschr 108:654–663

Weber U, Lüdtke R, Friese KH, Fischer I, Moeller H (2002) A non-randomized pilot study to compare complementary and conventional treatments of acute sinusitis. Forschende Komplementärmedizin 9:99–104

Weil RS (1997) Der hustende Patient in der hausärztlichen Praxis. Ther Erfolg 1:145–146

Weiser M, Clasen P (1994) Randomisierte plazebokontrollierte Doppelblindstudie zur Untersuchung der klinischen Wirksamkeit der homöopathischen Euphorbium compositum-Nasen-tropfen S bei chronischer Sinusitis. Forschende Komplementärmedizin 1:251–259

Weiser M Clasen P (1995) Controlled double-blind study of a homeopathic sinusitis medication. Biol Ther 13:4–11

White A, Slade P, Hunt C, Hart A, Ernst E (2003) Individualized homeopathy as an adjunct in the treatment of childhood asthma: a randomized, placebo controlled trial. Thorax 58:317–321

Wiesenauer M, Gaus W (1985) Double-blind trial comparing the effectiveness of the homeopathic preparation galphimia potency D6, galphimia dilution 10^{-6} and placebo on pollinosis. Arzneimittelforschung 35:1745–1747

Wiesenauer M, Gaus W, Bohnacker U, Haussler S (1989) Efficiency of homeopathic preparation combinations in sinusitis. Results of a randomized double-blind study with general practitioners. [in German]. Arzneimittelforschung 39:620–625

Zentralinstitut für kassenärztliche Versorgung in der Bundesrepublik Deutschland (ZKV) (1998) Die EVaS Studie. Wissenschaftliche Reihe, vol 39.1. Deutscher ÄrzteVerlag, Cologne

Safety of Homeopathic Use

Klaus v. Ammon, André Thurneysen

11.1   Introduction

With regard to unexpected side effects (adverse drug effects) it is necessary to distinguish between the ones which are characteristic to homeopathy and even intended and the known pharmacological-toxic effects of (otherwise appropriate) medicines.

Homeopathic medicines are expertly manufactured according to international pharmacopoeias (HAB 2000). High potencies are administered at sufficiently long intervals (cf. Chap. 3). The application of toxic primary substances in low potencies, especially as part of complexes, must be well-researched and safety-checked. To what extent sensible recommendations are always strictly observed is not known.

Supporters of homeopathy continue to insist that it has no side effects; a claim that is not unchallenged (see Oepen and Schaffrath 1993, p 265).

Toxic effects and adverse organ effects of drugs can almost be ruled out with expert prescription. They are different from the (typical) reactions which occur in (sensitive) individuals as part of homeopathic drug-proving or in ultra-sensitive patients during ordinary therapy as proving symptoms. Adverse reactions can be caused through incorrect application such as dosage repetition in too quick succession.

11.2   Responses to Treatment

An initial reaction at the functional level is possible following an individualized homeopathic prescription with high potencies even if it was given by a qualified practitioner. It can be strong enough to cause what is called 'initial aggravation' and can, in extreme cases, provoke the symptoms of a typical drug-proving. The return of old symptoms and skin reactions (which is in fact desirable) is seen as indicating an elimination process as described in Hering's Law of Cure. Frequency and severity of these reactions depend on various factors and do not constitute a problem with expertly delivered homeopathy.

If very low potencies are used unprofessionally, systemic toxic effects can occur (e.g. of arsenic, lead and mercury) similar to those known from pharmacology. The use of mother tinctures, which really belong to phytotherapy, can also result in topical or systemic symptoms of poisoning (Cardinali et al. 2004).

An isopathy study mentioned up to 24% initial aggravations (Reilly et al. 1986) which were probably caused by too-frequent drug dosages. Specific adverse drug reactions which decreased with repeated administration occurred in an influenza prevention study in 10% of patients compared with 2% unspecific complaints for placebo (Attena et al. 1995).

If homeopathic substances are taken as standard combinations (complex homeopathy) or simultaneously ('proven indication', clinical homeopathy), it is not possible to determine, and thus avoid, the component causing the adverse reaction.

Any homeopathic remedies, if incompetently applied by a qualified or lay person, can cause suppressions and adversely affect the course of the disease (cf. Chap. 3). Systematic assessment and confirmation of such findings are particularly difficult to achieve and have, to our knowledge, not yet been published.

11.3 Interaction of Substances

Some substances and medicines can inhibit, block or counteract homeopathic treatment (Sankaran 1984, Seider 1999). There is only anecdotal evidence of aggravating interactions (diphtheria serum, Hess 1942).

11.4 Safety of Application

The question of interactions of homeopathic treatment with allopathic medicines (hormones, antibiotics, cytostatics etc.) is frequently asked and can lead to a reluctance to prescribe these medicines. Homeopathic physicians carefully consider such situations and act in accordance with the general guidelines of medical responsibility. In practice it hardly ever happens that a homeopathic remedy has an adverse influence on the effect of allopathic drugs, while the effect of homeopathic treatment is clearly impaired by allopathic medicines.

11.5 Scientific Research

There are only few publications which demonstrate adverse effects, or unexpected adverse events (UAE), in general; a causal connection with the medication is not yet implied. A meta-analysis of 3437 patients from 24 placebo-controlled RCTs showed (only) 63 UAEs (1.54%) for patients treated with homeopathic remedies and 50 for placebo (1.45%). It concluded that there was no clear evidence of homeopathic initial aggravations (Grabia and Ernst 2003).

A summarising review was presented by Dantas and Rampes (2003), who found, on the basis of reports, an adverse event rate of 9.4% for homeopathic remedies as opposed to 6.1% with placebo, describing them as comparable, rare and transient. The authors deplore the low methodological quality of the publications.

The following investigations summarize single cases: Hentschel et al. (1998) reported that 63 (1.9%) of 3447 patients were treated homeopathically while in intensive care; 25 of them (39.7%), who had no pathological findings, thought their complaints were due to the homeopathic treatment. In nine of these cases conventional and homeopathic diagnosis and treatment were adequately documented. The authors recommend central registration as with conventional medicines.

IIPCOS (International Integrative Primary Care Outcomes Study) mentions a total of 8.3% of adverse events, which a third of the patients classified as 'strong'; half of these withdrew from the study and received therapeutic intervention. A causal connection with the investigational medication was assumed in only 3.4%. Intensity was rated 'medium' by half of these patients, and a quarter each described it as 'light' and 'severe', causing three patients to withdraw from the study and another three to seek other therapeutic measures (Heger et al. 2001).

Güthlin et al. (2004) showed that physicians reported fewer UAEs than patients did and assumed that physicians and patients interpret initial reactions differently.

Dantas and Rampes (2003) explain anecdotal reports of adverse effects in conventional medical journals with products that were not genuine homeopathic remedies but were wrongly referred to as 'homeopathic'.

A systematic search for individual cases in the homeopathic and legal literature was not possible owing to problems of infrastructure, methodology and time.

11.6   Safety: Summary and Conclusion

Medical homeopathy in Switzerland has few side effects if professionally executed, and the use of medium and high potencies is free from toxic and unexpected organ effects.

11.7   References

Attena F, Toscano G, Agozzino E, Del Giudice N (1995) A randomized trial in the prevention of influenza-like syndromes by homeopathic management. Rev Epidémiol Santé Publique 43:380–382

Cardinali C, Francalanci S, Giomi B, Caproni M, Sertoli A, Fabbri P (2004) Contact dermatitis from Rhus toxicodendron in a homeopathic remedy. J Am Acad Dermatol 50:150–151

Dantas F, Rampes H (2000) Do homeopathic medicines provoke adverse effects? A systematic review. Br Homeopathic J 89 [Suppl 1]:S35–38

Grabia S, Ernst E (2003) Homeopathic aggravations: a systematic review of randomized, placebo-controlled clinical trials. Homeopathy 92:92–98

Güthlin C, Lange O, Walach H (2004) Measuring the effects of acupuncture and homeopathy in general practice: an uncontrolled prospective documentation approach. BMC Public Health 4:6

Heger M, Riley DS, Haidvogl, Gordon D, Herrick N, Wolschner U, Thurneysen A (2001) IIPCOS – Ein internationales Projekt zur Untersuchung der Effektivität der Homöopathie in der ärztlichen Primärversorgung. HomInt R&D Newslett 2:3-19+27

Hentschel C, Kohnen R, Hahn EG (1998) Reports of complications in homeopathic treatment. In: Ernst E, Hahn EG (eds) Homeopathy – a critical appraisal. Butterworth, Oxford

Hess FO (1942) Nützt uns die Homöopathie bei der Diphtherie-Behandlung? Munchener Med Wochenschr 13:296

Oepen I, Schaffrath B (1993) Kritische Argumente zur Homöopathie. In: Oepen I (eds) Unkonventionelle medizinische Verfahren. Gustav Fischer, Stuttgart, Jena

Reilly DT, Taylor MA, McSharry C, Aitchison T Is homeopathy a placebo response? Lancet 1986 2:881–886

Sankaran P (1984) The clinical relationship of homeopathic remedies. The Homeopathic Medical Publishers, Bombay

Seider I (1999) Das kleine Buch der Arzneimittelbeziehungen. Barthel & Barthel, Starnberg

11

Cost-effectiveness
of Homeopathy

Klaus v. Ammon, René Gasser, Gudrun Bornhöft,
Stefanie Maxion-Bergemann

12.1   Introduction

Surveys conducted in the Western world all show that health-care costs tend to rise faster than general living costs. In the USA they rose from US$ 141 per person per year in 1960 through US$ 341 in 1970, US$ 1052 in 1980, and US$ 2689 in 1990 to US$ 4094 in 1998. For Switzerland the per person health-care costs were US$ 2412 in 1998 (see ◘ Fig. 12.2) and for Germany US$ 2222. All in all, the USA spent US$ 1100 billion on health care in 1998, Switzerland US$ 37 billion (see ◘ Fig. 12.1). In 2003, these costs rose to US$ 40 billion in Switzerland (CHF SFR 50 billion). They make up 11% (Swiztzerland) to 14% (USA) of the gross domestic product (cf. ◘ Fig. 12.3).

The overall costs for complementary medicine in Switzerland are estimated at 100–200 million CHF SFR (santésuisse), which is equivalent to 0.2 to –0.5% of all registered annual health-care costs (ca. 50 billion CHF SFR for 2003). (Data source: Bundesamt für Statistik[1], Switzerland, 2003).

Health-care expenditures that make up as high a percentage of the gross national product (GNP) as in the Western world are not sustainable in poor countries. Chile therefore recognized homeopathy at the end of the 19th century and permitted self-dispensing for by physicians. The Nigerian military government included homeopathy into its 1961 Medicare programme. In India homeopathy has been recognized since 1930, and it has been equivalent to Ayurveda and Western medicine since 1979. Romania publically recognized homeopathy in 1969. Brazil has accepted homeopathy as a 'medical subject' since 1979, but it has remained a privilege of the middle and upper classes. Cuba adopted homeopathy from Spain in 1845 and incorporated it into its national health system in 1992. Since 1994 it has been a compulsory part of medical studies in the Ukraine; a university chair was established in Kiev in 1992. In Malaysia, the ho-

---

1   Swiss Federal Statistical Office

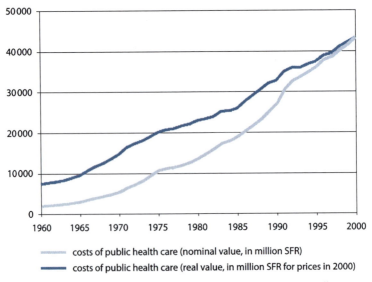

◘ Fig. 12.1 Health-care costs 1960–2000, in million SFR (source: Swiss Federal Statistical Office, 2003)

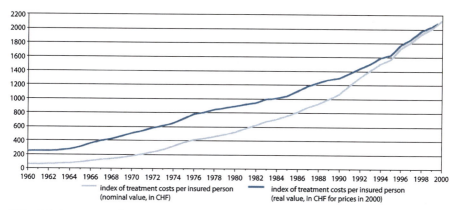

Fig. 12.2 Average costs of treatment per insured person and year, 1960–2000, in SFR (source: Swiss Federal Statistical Office 2003)

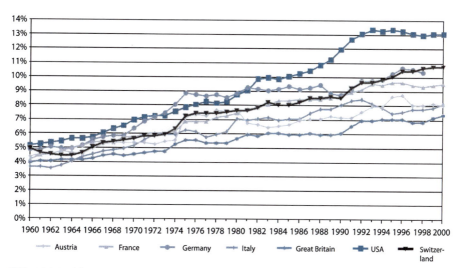

Fig. 12.3 Health-care costs in selected countries in % of gross domestic product from 1960 (source: Swiss Federal Statistical Office, 2003)

meopathic medical school, which was founded in 1979, became part of the university in 1996. In Mexico non-medical practitioners are on a par with qualified physicians. In Central and South America (Costa Rica, Venezuela, Columbia, Uruguay) recognition is only granted to qualified physicians. In Russia the recognition of homeopathy is being discussed by the Ministry of Health; Israel is preparing for recognition with a homeopathic outpatient clinic (Tel Aviv) and through clinical research (Hadassah Hospital, Jerusalem) (Schmidt 2001).

Exponentially rising health-care costs are hardly sustainable for strong economies either, and they are looking for ways to reduce the financial burden by investigating the efficacy, appropriateness and cost-effectiveness of certain medical systems.

12.2   Methods of Health Economics

For the health economic analysis of complementary medical approaches (as in the PEK project) the same methods can be used as for conventional health care.

Various health economic methods are available:

1. Cost-benefit analysis: relation of treatment costs to savings made due to the treatment, calculated in monetary units
2. Cost-effectiveness analysis: relation of treatment costs (in monetary units) to clinical benefit (e.g. complications avoided and years of life gained)
3. Cost-utility analysis
4. Cost-minimisation analysis

Costs are divided into:

1. direct costs: costs that arise from the illness itself, often separated into primary and secondary costs
2. indirect costs: inability to work, pensioning
3. intangible costs: quality of life (cannot be primarily expressed in monetary terms)

In order to ascertain the cost-effectiveness of a particular method it is necessary to assess, apart from its clinical effectiveness, also that of a comparable treatment in order to demonstrate real differences. If no such data are available, comparison of costs before and after the introduction of the method in question can also provide information as to whether costs have been reduced or increased. A number of influences have to be considered in the process that can also affect costs during the period of observation, such as the increasing age of observed patients, the general rise in health-care costs etc.

In order to assess the effectiveness of a clinical procedure, one can collect new (or primary) data or published (or secondary) data, or one can carry out new calculations on the basis of existing data (model calculations).

The method seen as the *sine qua non* in knowledge acquisition in clinical studies, the randomized, double-blind trial, can be applied only with reservations in health economics. The factors known to ensure a good RCT design also reduce its validity in actual practice reality. Yet it is the in actual practice reality where economic considerations must apply; and therefore data need to be assessed that are practice-relevant, or, if data from clinical studies are used, they need to be commented or adjusted accordingly.

Next to the efficacy of a method, its cost-effectiveness for the health-care system in question needs to be established, as systems, reimbursement and costs can vary considerably from one country to the next. If there are no cost data it is best to evaluate cost-effectiveness on the basis of resource consumption. This information is available in 'natural' units and allows for comparisons between methods, such as medicine consumption, consultation times etc. and can often be found among the results of clinical studies.

The definition of 'complementary medical methods' or complementary and alternative medicine (CAM), (complementary and alternative medicine) varies from study to study with regard to aspects such as products, treatment and activities. The version most frequently quoted in epidemiological studies is by Eisenberg et al. (1993, 1998): 'Interventions neither taught widely in medical schools nor generally available in the US hospitals'. Depending on the definition used, statements concerning the prevalence of CAM use also vary (Furler et al. 2003) and are therefore not directly comparable. The same is true for cost data: they can be compared only if they relate to the same, clearly defined intervention.

Although opinions concerning the exact number and definition of complementary medical methods differ, most authors distinguish 11 main disciplines: acupuncture, chiropractic, creative and sensory therapies, healing, phytotherapy, homeopathy, hypnosis, manual therapies, reflexology and osteopathy (Andrews et al. 2003).

Despite these difficulties, we provide here an overview of various surveys and studies on complementary therapies that include information on costs. In doing so, we not only document the current state of research on these topics, but also the problems that arise from the interpretation of results. If nothing else, they can serve to generate further, more clearly defined research questions and underline the importance of a clear delimitation to other approaches and providers.

12.3 Use of CAM

In the 1990s, major studies detected trends towards the use of alternative and complementary medical methods in the USA (Eisenberg et al. 1993 and 1998). In 1990 almost 34% of Americans interviewed reported that they had used at least one CAM treatment in the year preceding the interview; in 1997 this percentage rose to 46.3 % of interviewees ($p=0.002$). The number of CAM users who paid for the treatment 'out of pocket' hardly changed (from 64.0% to 58.3%).

The prevalence of CAM use in Canada was between 15% and 52% in 1996 and 1997, with a 20% increase since 1992 (Furler et al. 2003). Estimated out-of-pocket spending on CAM was CA\$ 3.8 million in 1996/97 (US\$ 2.4 million).

In Ontario, the consumption of natural medical products (vitamins, minerals, food supplements, herbs, homeopathy and other CAM products) rose from 16% to 33% between 1998 and 2001 (Furler et al. 2003).

Interviews and surveys done in Germany and the UK revealed that complementary medical methods were used parallel to conventional ones (Thomas et al. 2001, Dixon et al. 2003), but the data do not allow for conclusions to be drawn regarding overall costs. It is not at all rare for patients to consult different physicians. This can be compared to the simultaneous use of home remedies and specialized medical treatment.

Various studies showed that, in the UK, CAM supply and demand have grown considerably in recent years (Andrews et al. 2003). Fisher and Ward (1994) demonstrated that up to 25% of the population use complementary medicine each year (cf. Vickers 1994); Thomas et al. (2001) estimated that 33% of the population used CAM in one form or another at least once in their lifetime.

The Swiss health surveys of 1997 and 2002 did not find evidence of a significant rise in provision by homeopathic physicians after inclusion of their therapy method into the national health insurance catalogue (KVG[2]), which also speaks for a currently subsidiary use of homeopathy in Switzerland and contradicts the quasi-experimental approach of the study of Sommer et al. (1999); cf. also Chap. 8.

For more information on the use of CAM in Switzerland see Chap. 8;, for international use see Chap. 7.

---

2   KVG – Krankenversicherungsgesetz

12.4 Costs

In a cost appraisal one needs to differentiate the perspective from which the calculation is carried out (that of the insurer, physician or patient), as amounts vary accordingly. When there are additional costs to pay for the patient, the physician has to take his practice costs as a basis, the health insurer the services that have to be reimbursed. There are also different kinds of costs: direct costs (caused by the illness), indirect costs (e.g. days off work, premature pensioning) and intangible costs (not directly measurable in monetary units, quality-of-life aspects). By comparing the costs incurred through different interventions, potential savings can be established.

Direct costs for homeopathy include consultation and repertorisation. They are listed in the *tarif médicale* (TARMED) just like laboratory and instrument examinations. The medicines prescribed are listed in a pharmaceutical speciality index (Spezialitätenliste: SL) and are fully reimbursed.

Other direct costs are not specific to homeopathy and include expert consultations, referrals to colleagues and specialists in complementary or conventional medicine in private practice or hospitals for diagnosis and (in- or outpatient) treatment. For expert consultations and referrals they can be centrally assessed through TARMED (swissmédic) and new-index (Trustcenter). Indirect costs arise through sick leave (incapacity to work) and invalidity.

Homeopathic therapy also offers saving opportunities by avoiding other prescriptions: the potential savings for conventional medicines that are thrown away are estimated to be at least CHF SFR 2 billion (Breu 1999).

In the long term, patient satisfaction (Christen et al. 2000) could find expression in direct cost savings (e.g. unnecessary surgery, health resorts) and indirect cost savings (sick-leave compensation) (Güthlin et al. 2004). German pilot projects indicate a sustainable effect with complementary medical methods (see Sect. 12.11).

12.5 Cost-effectiveness

It must always be possible to establish the cost-effectiveness of a method by looking at how the costs relate to the benefits. The benefit can be found through clinical studies, economic data are either gathered directly with the clinical study, in a later survey or with a model calculation. Information about the consumption or savings of resources can support the evaluation if no cost data are available. With complementary medical specialities, the quality of life must also be assessed, because it is an important parameter in the evaluation of a method's effectiveness.

In legal terms, the necessity for economy extends to all aspects of the medical treatment including consultation costs, analyses, expert consultation, application and prescription of medicines and, in the widest sense, the costs of hospitaliszation, health resorts, incapacity to work and invalidity (Art. 25 § 2, KVG[3], Switzerland). These costs can be established systematically by comparing average costs (KSK[4] statistics) or by analysing single case reports. The latter can compensate for the known shortcomings of the KSK treatment case statistics. TARMED's new tariff structure (1 January 2004) offers the possibility to carry out such surveys via 'Trust Centres', independently of the billing statistics of santésuisse (alliance of Swiss health insurers,

---

3   Krankenversicherungsgesetz – Swiss Health Insurance Act
4   Konkordat der Schweizerischen Krankenkassen – Swiss Health Insurance Association

formerly KSK). Especially with single case assessments it is possible to take into account compensatory savings as special features that are particularly effective in practice.

12.6 Reimbursement

The demand for CAM has risen continuously in recent years and, as shown by various studies and surveys, at a similar rate in different countries (Eisenberg et al. 1998). The health services therefore ask which therapies should be reimbursed. Pelletier (2002) conducted a survey to investigate coverage of costs by insurance providers and other health-care payers. Based on telephone interviews with hospitals and insurance companies and an extensive literature research, he came to the following conclusions: indication for a medical intervention was a necessary condition for reimbursement. Reasons for the decision in favour of reimbursing complementary medical therapies were (in order of importance): market research, retention of members, demand by members or consumers, incentive for new members, demand by providers/companies, possible savings, possibly less invasive etc. It is noticeable that the wishes of potential clients play an important part in the decision-making process, while scientific aspects are less important.

A publication by Conrad et al. (1998) investigated the extent to which treatment decisions of physicians are influenced by reimbursement/payment considerations. They assessed therapy costs, number of consultations and hospital days in relation to the reimbursement method (direct payment without 'service incentives'; over 50% basic compensation plus service incentives; over 50% dependent on service provided + further service incentives; only dependent only on service provided; other methods). The authors interviewed 865 physicians (Washington) and found no significant correspondence between the kind of compensation (how the physician was paid) and the treatment decision.

12.7 Data and Studies for Homeopathy

The first (tendentious) cost-benefit analysis in favour of homeopathy was published by Bradford (1900) on the basis of reports collected in Europe and the USA since 1850, on mortalities, and with cost comparisons.

Several recent epidemiological examinations have developed models that register all direct and indirect costs of homeopathy and partly compare them with other treatment methods (Heger et al. 2001, Riley et al. 2001, Becker-Witt et al. 2003; Güthlin et al. 2001).

Cost comparisons aim at minimising the total costs while retaining at least equal effectiveness measured, for instance, in days of work and consumption of analgesics, and benefit measured in specific outcome or improvement of co-morbidities with financial advantages such as reduced health insurance premiums. This was investigated in a study which also demonstrated, by way of example, that patients are willing to contribute to health costs with up to 20% of their income in order to cure their arthritis (White et al. 1996).

The following studies assessed specific overall costs:

The international prospective outcome study IIPCOS-1 with 348 patients in 6 six centres (in Germany, Austria, Switzerland and the USA) used the Glasgow Homeopathic Hospital (GHH) outcome scale and found an 80.5% improvement of complaints after two 2 weeks of treatment (Heger et al. 2001).

There is a national prospective observational study for Germany (100 physicians + 4 four physicians from Switzerland) comparing homeopathy and acupuncture (Becker-Witt et al. 2004), one for homeopathy in Belgium (van Wasserhoven & and Ives 2004) and two for France (Chaufferin 2000, Trichard et al. 2003). For India or Cuba no studies are currently known to us.

There is a local overview for Glastonbury (Hills and Welford 2003) and Newcastle (Soloman 2003 quoted from Slade et al. 2004) in Britain.

A regional overview of homeopathy arose out of an investigation launched by the German health insurer IKK[5] (Güthlin et al. 2004). A systematic nationwide survey for Germany was published in the *Gesundheitsberichterstattung des Bundes*[6] (Marstedt & and Moebus 2002, see also Sect. 12.11 below).

There are also studies which focus on indications: the IIPCOS[7] studies (Heger et al. 2000, Heger et al. 2001, Riley et al. 2001) and individual studies on female infertility, rheumatoid arthritis, otitis media, atopies and allergies, dyspepsia and asthma. The direct costs saved on average for infertility are almost unbelievable (ca. 335 vs. 11,661.50 DM). In addition to that, conventionally treated women are hospitalized six times as often (Gerhard et al. 1993).

The only patient collectives investigated so far are children: De Lange de Klerk et al. (1994) noted fewer recurrences and a lower antibiotics consumption of antibiotics with homeopathy; Frei and Thurneysen (2001) examined children with otitis media, Keil (2001) children with allergies, Frenkel and Hermoni (2002) children with atopies, and Junker et al. (2004) children with dystonia.

▫ Table 12.3 lists more clinical studies that demonstrated shorter duration of illness and reduced consumption of conventional medicines due to homeopathic treatment.

An international study in Germany and Austria on specialist physician groups gives evidence that in primary health care each per cent of improvement under homeopathic treatment costs half as much as under conventional medical treatment (Haidvogl et al. 2001). In analogy to regional investigations from Britain (Swayne 1992) the German *Kassenärztliche Vereinigung* (association of statutory health insurance physicians) in Northern Wurttemberg showed for the second quarter of 1988 the same direct physician provision, but statistically significant differences (15%) for medication and sick leave certificates with 97 general and 87 naturopathic practitioners or homeopaths, corresponding to overall savings of 8.2%. The German Hahnemann Society published an article in the medical journal *Ärzteblatt* (15/1989) in Lower Saxony with the title 'Homeopaths work more cost-effectively'. Dentists were investigated retrospectively (therefore not randomized) with regard to the cost benefits homeopathy has for insured persons: Feldhaus (1993) demonstrated that Arnica C12 reduced the rate of complications and sick leave certificates by 40%, resulting in savings of DM 1209 per patient and year in direct costs alone.

Investigations are rarely performed in hospitals: Van Haselen (2000) conducted a cost study at the Royal London Homeopathic Hospital; in Clover (2000) a cost analysis is missing.

For single cases, costs have so far mostly been documented only in the context of legal action, either on behalf of the patient or the physician.

It is certainly possible to demonstrate that (individual) homeopathic physicians work on average (clearly) more economically than their colleagues in conventional medicine: 'A child psychiatrist who works almost exclusively with homeopathy considerably lowers the average

---

5   Innungskrankenkasse – German health insurance provider
6   federal health service report
7   International Integrative Primary Care Outcomes Study

cost compared with other specialists' (Gmür 2003). In 1988/89 the direct costs charged by a homeopathic paediatrician to the statutory health services was were more than 50% below the average in his specializsation group. His hospital referrals were also below the average of comparable conventional physicians. Homeopaths generate only 1560–1560% of the drug costs of their conventional colleagues. In addition, there are basically no costs caused by side effects. The same is true for prevalently homeopathic treatment in hospitals (Drähne 1991). It is possible in Switzerland, due to TARMED (santésuisse and new-index for the assessment of cost neutrality and of 'physician ratings'), and it was also possible in Germany up to 1997, due to regional associations of statutory health insurance physicians, to keep data relating to individual physicians and physician groups (see above) confidential.

From the point of view of health insurance providers, the EGK-SVHA[8] Family Physician System has achieved, since 1 January 1997, i.e. within three 3 years, premium reductions of ca. 10% for patients, good compensation for physicians (CHF SFR 200 per hour in 5-minute slots, similar to the later TARMED 2004 regulations), and at least an initial, small net gain for the health insurer (Müller 2000). At the end of 2003 this interesting model expired due to conditions set by the regulator.

Summary

In terms of cost economics, the initially higher direct costs for physicians in homeopathy are certainly balanced out (Becker-Witt et al. 2003, Hills and Welford 2004). They are even undercut due to the reduced costs for laboratory and technical services and due to lower indirect costs accrued through sick leave and invalidity, especially in the long term (Güthlin et al. 2004, Slade et al. 2004).

12.8 Data and Projects from Switzerland

More data concerning the use of complementary medical therapies can be found in Chaps. 7 and 8.

The period during which five CAM disciplines were provisionally included in the Swiss statutory health insurance (1999 - 2005) has been largely evaluated, as have the PEK data (cf. Chapter 1, Introduction). The results of this evaluation confirm the cost-effectiveness of CAM [Studer and Busato 2010, 2011]. From 2012 all five CAM methods will be re-included in the Swiss statutory health insurance for a further provisional period of six years.

12.8.1 NFP 34

Between 1993 and 1998, the NFP[9] 34 was carried out in Switzerland on various complementary medical topics including a study on health economics.

Sommer et al. (1999) conducted an experimental study which investigated the economic consequences of including complementary medical therapies in the statutory health care provi-

---

8   EGK: Eidgenössische Gesundheitskasse – Swiss Federal Health Insurance
    SVHA: Schweizerischer Verein Homöopatischer Ärztinnen und Ärzte – Swiss Association of Homeopathic
    Physicians
9   NFP Nationales Forschungsprogramm – National Research Program

sion for a part of the insured persons compared with members without this extra benefit and members paying voluntary additional insurance contributions. In a randomiszed procedure, 7682 clients of the biggest largest Swiss insurer, Helvetia, were offered free use of complementary medical therapies for three 3 years (1993–1995). The other clients (670,000) presented constituted the control group and were divided into the subgroups 'without this benefit' and 'with voluntary additional insurance'.

For the assessment of the economic effect, cost data and – in a smaller group – data on life quality were collected in questionnaire SF-36.

The following questions were asked:
1. Are complementary medical services that are paid for by the health insurer used as an addition to or instead of orthodox treatment?
2. What costs or savings are incurred by including complementary medicine into the statutory health provision?
3. How does the inclusion of complementary medicine into the statutory health provision affect the health of insured persons?

The results show that only 6.6% of the insured took advantage of the additional offer. Neither the costs nor the SF-36 data pointed to significant changes. Further analyses conducted by the authors revealed that less than 1% of the insured persons had used only complementary medicine.

The mean costs for complementary medicine per insured person were CHF SFR 1 per head before project start (1992); by 1995 they had risen to CHF SFR 30 in the experimental group and to CHF SFR 18 in the group without additional insurance. The costs for conventional medical treatment were CHF SFR 1366 in 1992 (experimental group) and CHF SFR 1358 (control group), rising to CHF SFR 1857 (experimental group) and CHF SFR 1840 (control group) by 1995.

The state of health of the insured slightly deteriorated during the observation period, presumably because of the growing increasing age of the group. Analysis of the individual groups showed that the state of health of the insured persons who paid voluntary additional insurance contributions and of those who had cost-free additional insurance (experimental group) was significantly worse than that of patients without additional insurance.

The authors draw the overall conclusion that reimbursement for complementary medicine by the statutory health services neither leads neither to cost containment nor to health benefits.

The publication of these study results and the conclusions drawn from them fuelled a broad public debate. (Heusser 1999, Kiene & and Kiene 1999, Studer 1999). Points of criticism mostly related to structural aspects and questioned the conclusions drawn by the authors from their collection of data. Especially the conclusion concerning additive usage does not follow from the available data. More details on the discussion follow below (Sect. 12.12).

12.8.2 Further data from Switzerland

The diploma thesis by Bolis (2003), which evaluates the outcome of the 1997 and 2002 Swiss Health Survey and was published recently as part of the PEK project, came to the following conclusions with regard to homeopathy: 'The [...] analysis shows that the average number of physician consultations in general, i.e. without differentiation of the kind of treatment delivered (conventional or homeopathic), was significantly higher for patients who had used homeopathy in the previous 12 months (5.4 consultations per year) than for the overall population (4.4 consultations per year). The same patients see physicians who practice only conventional medicine, significantly less frequently (2.2 consultations per year on average) than the overall population (4.4); and only 20% of homeopathy users see only homeopathically trained physicians. Until a more in-depth study is available, one can conclude that homeopathy is seen mostly as complementary to allopathic medicine while being used as a substitute in some cases.'

More data on Switzerland can be found in the statistics of the Swiss Federal Statistical Office Health Survey 1997 and 2002.

12.9   International CAM Studies and Surveys: Patients

International publications were also evaluated to assess the costs of alternative healing approaches. There are 15 publications in total that include the cost situation of various countries: Australia (3), Canada (1), Germany (3), UK (3) and USA (5). All of these publications investigated the use of CAM in general, which means that the information given does not relate to a particular method but shows the frequency and quantity of CAM usage for various approaches: mostly all the kinds of therapies that are not prescribed by conventional physicians.

The data are not really comparable, as costs are stated in different units and different services (which are mostly not clearly defined) were used.

The costs for these treatments are usually not reimbursed in the countries named and are referred to as 'out-of-pocket' spending, which means that the patient pays for them himself.

Only two publications state that the National Health Service (NHS) in the UK reimbursed 10% (Thomas et al. 2001) and the insurance in the USA ca. 30% (von Grueningen et al. 2001).

When the cost of CAM usage is assessed, one often evaluates services that are fundamentally different: physician-led treatments with prescription medicines and over-the-counter (OTC) medication. We therefore do not list publications here that show overall costs, because information on costs is either too imprecise or absent (MacLennan et al. 1996; Rees et al. 2000; Fairfield et al. 1998; Patterson et al. 2002).

The costs shown below relate to only one therapy (e.g. TCM therapy as a whole – traditional Chinese medicine – for one particular indication). Treatment costs per patient and month were between A$ 7 (Australia; Buchbinder et al. 2002) and A$ 66 (Australia, Shenfield et al. 2002), between CA$ 0 and 250 (Canada, Furler et al. 2003) and £ 13.62 with a standard deviation of £ 1.61 (UK, Ernst and White 2000).

Other publications show costs per treatment and patient without mentioning a time frame: € 205 (ranging from €15 to €1278) in Germany (Schäfer et al. 2002), US$ 414 ± US$ 269 (Egede et al. 2002) and US$ 1127 (Ramsay et al. 2001) in the USA.

Most publications also include statements on the frequency of CAM use next to those on costs. The resulting figures differ depending on the questioning method, the population investigated and the definition of CAM that was used: The range of general CAM usage varies between 10.6% (UK, Thomas et al. 2001: asking about CAM usage in year before survey) and 77% (Canada, Furler et al. 2003: asking about current use). The figures for individual therapies are as follows: phytotherapy ('herbalist'): 5.4 % (Australia, Shenfield et al. 2002), 0.4% (Australia, MacLennan et al. 1996); 3.8%, 95% CI: 2.5–5.5 (UK, Rees et al. 2000); homeopathy: 32% (Australia, Shenfield et al. 2002); 1.2% (Australia, MacLennan et al. 1996); 1.85%, 95% CI: 1.0–3.1 (UK, Rees et al. 2000).

Despite the lack of comparability of data, the results prove that the costs of CAM therapies are relatively low. If one assumes a comparable effect with other therapeutic measures, one can at least not expect an increase of costs with CAM therapies.

12.10 **International CAM Studies and Surveys on: Physicians/Providers**

The first study to deal with CAM providers was conducted in the UK by Burton and the Osteopathy Association of Great Britain (Andrews et al. 2003). It focused mainly on the structure of osteopathy practices, especially on the age and experience of the therapists.

A literature review by Astin et al. (1998) also indicates that a high number of conventional physicians are in favour of complementary medical methods and therefore either refer patients or apply complementary medical methods themselves. On average, 16% of physicians said that they used herbal medicines and 9% that they used homeopathy. The investigation showed that average referrals to a CAM specialist were 43% for acupuncture and 4% for herbal medicine.

The authors pointed out, however, that the study designs were very different and the data therefore not comparable. They nevertheless conclude that there is, in general, a high percentage of physicians who either use CAM or refer patients to CAM specialists.

12.11 **Pilot Projects in Germany**

In order to investigate alternative diagnosis and healing methods, health insurance providers in Germany are entitled to conduct pilot projects. As part of these projects, members are, under certain conditions, granted treatments which are not included among the benefits of the *Gesetzliche Krankenversicherung* (GKV[10]). ◻ Table 12.4 lists the individual projects. Most of them focus on chronically ill patients, and the methods offered are partly restricted to acupuncture and homeopathy. The observation studies are purely descriptive in structure and belong therefore to the field of provision research. Their main objectives are to show procedures in close connection to the actual practice, to identify trends, and to acquire knowledge on economic effects. The projects cannot provide the kind of evidence of effectiveness that is supplied by clinical studies.

The investigations aim at assessing and evaluating the following data (with differences depending on the project): use, drug prescriptions, incapacity to work, state of health and satisfaction.

First results of individual projects (interim analyses) have now been published:

I. Project of the *Betriebskrankenkassen* (BKK[11]): various CAM therapies (Moebus et al. 1998):
To investigate various CAM therapies, 21 *Betriebskrankenkassen* in total conducted a pilot project for chronically sick ill patients who had tried all conventional treatment options without success. From among a total of ca. 70,000 insured persons, 386 patients took part in the 2-year pilot phase. A first evaluation (ITT analysis) after 2 years showed the following results:
- Average duration of disease 10 years when starting pilot project.
- Differences between user and 'normal population': users take more exercise, are more concerned about their health, tend to think that they can influence their own state of health; state of health worse, stronger severity of symptoms.
- Days off work: a trend towards a decrease of days off work is registered after project start, but case numbers are too low to allow for definite conclusions.

---

10 Statutory Health Insurance (SHI)
11 Company health insurance providers

- Hospitalisation: costs reduced by 5.9%.
- Physician and dentist outpatient costs: assessment of 46 patients with treatment completed: 10fold tenfold increase in costs (short duration of pilot project needs to be considered).
- Overall costs: At the time of evaluation no comparison data were available; therefore no statement possible.
- Symptom analysis: reduction of symptom score by 40% within the first 3 months after treatment start, below 50% after 6 months, effect persisting after 18 months.

II. Project of the *Bundesverband der Innungskassen* (BV IKK[12]): acupuncture, homeopathy (Walach et al. 1997, Güthlin et al. 2001, Güthlin et al. 2004):
First figures are also available from another project: the examination of acupuncture and homeopathy by the health insurance companies IKK Saxony, IKK Saxony-Anhalt and IKK Baden-Württemberg in association with their federal association. The prospective study followed catamnesis over a period of 5 years with ca. 3000 patients using acupuncture and 1000 patients using homeopathy. All insurance members were allowed to take part in the project.
- The first analysis (ca. 110 patients evaluated, Walach et al. 1997) showed that around 50% of patients professed to be cured or clearly better after treatment.
- A second, later analysis (Güthlin et al. 2001) which evaluated data of ca. 1500 patients showed that more than 65% of homeopathically treated patients said they were clearly better or cured after 6 months. Estimations by physicians were comparable. 80% of patients were 'satisfied' with their treatment, which corresponds to the significant difference in quality of life (assessed with questionnaire MOS-SF36) before and after treatment.
- Days off work: no difference before and after treatment, but simultaneous rising trend in the overall population and mostly evaluation of chronically sick patients. The lack of change could therefore be seen as an advantage.

In the meantime, a final evaluation has been published (Güthlin et al. 2004) which reports the following results: A total of 5292 patients were treated with acupuncture and 933 with homeopathy; 53 patients received both. The figures reflect the ratio of providing physicians.
Results for acupuncture: When asked whether their complaints had improved under treatment 36% said they were 'a lot better', 49% 'better', and there was 'no change' for 13%; 1% said they were worse. In the estimation of the physicians the therapeutic effect showed an improvement by 0.9 points (standard deviation 0.5) on a 7-point scale. Regarding quality of life (SF-36) the greatest improvement was for 'bodily pain scale' and 'physical role'.
For the assessment of days off work, data from the last preceding 16 years were evaluated. They showed an increase of days before treatment and a decrease after. The patients who used CAM had a relatively high number of sick days per year at the beginning of the project (on average 32 days, standard deviation 67 days); 2–3 years into the pilot project they reached approximately the same level as the comparison group of non-CAM users (after 3 years: on average 13 days, standard deviation 14 days; after 5 years: on average 7 days, standard deviation 33 days). Before project begin CAM users had registered a steady increase in days off work from 8 days on average 6 years before the project to 32 days in the year when the project started.
Results for homeopathy: When asked whether their complaints had improved under treatment 39% said they were 'a lot better', 38% 'better', and there was 'no change' for 17%; 2% said they were worse. The estimation of the therapeutic effect by physicians showed an improvement

---

12 Federal association of guild health insurers

by 0.95 points (standard deviation 0.5) on a 7-point scale. With regard to the quality of life (SF-36) a substantial improvement was registered by 15–20% (absolute change, different depending on dimension of questionnaire SF-36, greatest improvement for 'physical role'), which persisted throughout the 30 months of observation.

With regard to the data on days off work, the data of the last 16 years were evaluated. They showed an increase in days off work before the treatment and a decrease after. The patients who used CAM, had an average of 19 sick days per year at the beginning of the project (standard deviation 48 days); 3 years into the pilot project the average reached had dropped to 13 days (standard deviation 40 days) and after 5 years the average was 11 days (standard deviation 52 days). Before the project started the patients of the CAM group registered a steady increase in days off work from an average of 8 days 6 years before project begin to 19 days in the year when it started.

III. Overall evaluation

An overall evaluation of data from the two first projects mentioned was conducted in 2001/2002 in the context of a federal health report (Marstedt and Moebus 2002). It showed the following results:

In both pilot projects, a definite and sustained decrease was noted in days off work in the before-after comparison, from initially 32 days to 23 (24) days in the second year of observation after treatment begin. The effects were stronger or manifested earlier for men. The authors concluded a health-economic significance of this sustained decrease (cf. also ◻ Table 12.1). The long-term days off work rate sank continuously. The percentage of employees without days off work in one observation year rose by 36% to 47% in the same period of time.

A sustained improvement of the general state of health, measured in terms of quality of life, was also observed.

◻ **Table 12.1** Changes in days off work in the course of the pilot project of German regional health insurers BKK Essen/Cologne and the federal association IKK/IKK Saxony-Anhalt (IKKN)

Year of observation	Sick day rate[1]		Days[2]	
	BKK	IKK	BKK	IKK
-3	66	59	23	22
-1	68	62	32	31
1	68	60	27	33
2	59	56	23	24
4	56	51	22	18

[1] Percentage of patients with one incident of sick leave in 1 year (%) (patients with more than one incident are not listed separately)
[2] Average per patient per observation year
Source: Marstedt & Moebus (2002)

12.12   Discussion

12.12.1   Methodology

The discussion on the extent to which complementary medical treatments can be reflected in conventional health economics terms is ongoing. (Eisebitt 1999, Schüppel 2003, Marx 1997). In principle it should be possible, but the special conditions surrounding the methods of complementary medicine must be considered. These include that the individual patient-physician relationship is maintained, that physician and patient are free in the choice of treatment, and that the patient groups to be examined are not selected, as this comes closer to the real-life situation.

In an overview by White et al. (1996) the various methods of health economics are introduced. The authors request the inclusion of further outcome parameters for the evaluation of effectiveness for complementary medical therapies such as quality of life, while pointing out that the discussion regarding the monetary evaluation of the quality of life remains inconclusive. A qualitatively valuable and transparent assessment of a method's clinical efficacy (best provided by a clinical study) is a definite prerequisite for the calculation of cost-effectiveness.

Buxton (UK, 2000) also concludes in his paper 'Assessing the cost-effectiveness of homeopathic medicines' that, regarding a realistic evaluation of a method's efficacy and cost-effectiveness, there is growing experience and understanding of the worth of large-scale, multi-centre, pragmatic (as opposed to explanatory and experimental) studies. NICE (National Institute for Clinical Excellence, UK) also supports the inclusion of 'good evidence' into the formal clinical guidelines in certain cases. The author further requests that not just clinical efficacy be measured in traditional units but that quality of life and patient preferences also be included in the evaluation of a treatment's effectiveness.

12.12.2   Cost-effectiveness of complementary medical methods

The publications regarding costs that are available in the field of complementary medicine can be divided into three categories:
1. Surveys of the prevalence of CAM use and costs arising from it
2. Surveys of pilot project data for the evaluation of quality-of-life parameters and costs arising from using CAM
3. Cost-effectiveness analyses on individual methods of complementary medicine

Data sources for the first two categories have the following restrictions regarding their appropriateness in evaluating the costs arising from the use of a specific complementary medical method:
1. All studies examine the simultaneous use of several CAM methods with – in some cases – very broad definitions of the CAM therapies under investigation.
2. The investigational populations vary from special patient groups with one indication (such as allergies or HIV) to spot-check interviews among the population.
3. A few studies have methodical shortcomings which render a comparison between users and non-users of CAM impossible.
4. Data collected on 'out-of-pocket' costs do not allow inference to the costs resulting from reimbursements of one or several complementary medical methods.

◨ Table 12.2 Homeopathy: health economics studies and other investigations

Author, year, title	Country	Method	Participant, diagnosis	
Bleul (1997) Kostenvergleich Homöopathie/ Konventionelle Medizin am Beispiel zweier Fälle von akutem Tinnitus	Germany	calculation of costs per case: comparison of homeopathic and allopathic medication	acute tinnitus	
Chaufferin (2000) Improving the evaluation of homeopathy: economic considerations and impact on health	France	**data collection** (health insurers, statistics etc.) + **evaluation:** cost of medication, costs/outpatient, total costs/ treatment, quantitative ratio of homeopathic therapies + **Ipsos-study:** survey of 946 persons	various data on the overall volume of medication and therapies of all specialities	
Heger et al. (2001) IIPCOS – Ein internationales Projekt zur Untersuchung der Effektivität der Homöopathie in der ärztlichen Primärversorgung	Germany, Austria, Switzerland, USA	prospective outcome study: comparison of homeopathic and conventional therapy; selection of therapy by investigating physician (who was qualified in homeopathy)	348 patients (upper and lower respiratory tract infection, allergies, injuries, teething problems, abdominal pain)	
Schlüren (1984) Vergleich der Arzneimittelkosten bei homöopathischer und allopathisch-schulmedizinischer Behandlung	Germany	Retrospective analysis of cost data on the use of medication on gynaecological wards. Comparison of homeopathic and allopathic wards (mean value of three wards)	costs of medicines over 5 years for all patients of various gynaecological wards	

▼

Results	Comments
cost per case (calculated for two cases from a practice based on the German *Gebührenordnung für Ärzte (GOÄ[1])*: **treatment costs** (HP-consultations)[2]: case 1: 642.50 DM (total time 2.26 h) case 2: 519.20 DM (total time 2.03 h) **cost of medication:** ■ homeopathic medicines (actual figures): 8.35 DM ■ allopathic medicines (estimated): 383 DM	The authors state that compensation for the work expended is about the same for conventional and for homeopathic treatment (due to fee schedule). There is an obvious difference for the cost of medication. If one considers the likely side effects of conventional treatment or the (often recommended) hospitalisation for tinnitus, further costs of up to 5000 DM can arise. Even with appropriate compensation for the time expended for homeopathic history-taking one can still assume definite cost savings compared to with conventional treatment.
data evaluation: **prices of medicines:** costs for homeopathic medicines are 1/5 or 1/4 that of allopathic ones (price refunded, sales price) **spending on medication[3]:** Health expenses caused by homeopathic physicians are 42% below those of general practitioners. Homeopathic physicians claim 38% less compensation for medical provisions, 45% less for medication and 68% fewer days off work. **Ipsos-study:** 87% of patients who used homeopathic treatment did not consult conventional care providers for this case/illness.	Homeopathic remedies amount to less than 1% of medicaments reimbursed in France. Problems with evaluating the data: ■ comparability of data from homeopathic and general practices is restricted, as the patients were different ■ frequent use of homeopathic remedies by conventional practices (evaluation according to practices is therefore problematic). The authors point out that cost-effectiveness as well as the kind of utilisation of the homeopathic therapy (additive, substitutive, exclusive) have to be clarified. They request more and better-designed trials on the cost-effectiveness of homeopathy.
response rate ('complaint-free' or 'definite improvement' after 14 days): 80.5% (Europe only: 90.1%) 84% of patients were treatable exclusively with homeopathy, 16% needed conventional treatment in addition (antibiotics in only 1.4% of all participants) average duration of consultation: 16 min	About half of the patients paid for their treatment themselves.
Cost of medication 1973–1977 (5 years, DM): ■ homeopathic ward: 72,313 DM ('blood replacement'[4]: 23,133 DM, specialties: 49,180 DM) ■ allopathic ward: 120,262 DM ('blood replacement': 39,865 DM, specialties: 80,397 DM) ■ overall difference: 47,949 DM.	With the same effectiveness, costs for medication are three times higher with conventional treatment than with homeopathic treatment. Restriction: comparability applies only when overall costs are considered. Good: the wards are comparable with regard to patients and physicians.

▣ **Table 12.2** (continued)

Author, year, title	Country	Method	Participant, diagnosis	
Swayne (1992) The cost and effectiveness of homeopathy	UK	pilot study: data collected from 20 physicians to compare various cost data for homeopaths and data from the same area.	22 general practitioners	
Taieb and Myon (2003) The economic impact of homeopathic management: the French example (ISPOR Abstract)	France	longitudinal, prospective observation study (6 months) comparing homeopathic and allopathic treatment:	300 patients, chronic rhinitis	
Thomas et al (2001) Use and expenditure on complementary medicine in England: a population based survey	UK	Post-questioning to assess use of and expenditure on CAM treatments. Here: results for homeopathy	5010 adults (stratified random sample)	
Trichard et al. (2003) (ISPOR Poster)	France	Prospective practice study, comparing homeopathic and allopathic treatments	394 patients, anxiety disorder[7]	
Van Haselen (2000). The economic evaluation of complementary medicine: a staged approach at the Royal London Homeopathic Hospital	UK	UK (Royal London Homeopathic Hospital): Pilot project to evaluate cost effectiveness of homeopathic treatment. All patients had had conventional treatment and started homeopathic treatment at the beginning of the evaluation period.	499 (retrosp.) + 70 (prosp.) patients with rheumatic disorders	

12

▼

Results	Comments
mean percentage of homeopathic consultations: 24% Comparison: homeopathic physicians/ data from the area: ■ mean number of prescriptions per patient: 0.536/0.612 ■ mean number of prescriptions per unit: 0.408/0.439 ■ mean costs per prescription/patient: £ 0.92 homeopathic medication/ £ 4.61 general practice	Despite the study's various shortcomings[5] there are clear indications of cost savings through homeopathy. The authors suggest aspects for further studies.
cost per patient after 3 months: ■ allopathic treatment: 45.74 € ■ homeopathic treatment: 27.0 €	30% cost reduction compared with allopathic treatment (with comparable effectiveness)
homeopathy: number of consultations/year [6]: 1.31 m. (projection for UK) cost per patient and treatment (mean value, out-of-pocket or reimbursed): £ 27.20	CAM was more likely to be used by younger patients and women. Annual costs (mostly out of pocket) for CAM estimated at £ 450 m; in comparison: NHS expenditure for treatments in the same year was £ 3,846 m (medication not included). The data disprove the assumption of Ernst et al. that the number of consultations is higher for CAM physicians than for GPs. The authors conclude that the data confirm the importance of CAM as a first access to primary health care and demand more research to investigate cost-effectiveness of individual methods and, if the outcome should suggest this, to establish access to treatment via the NHS.
direct costs/patient (medication, consultation, tests, perspective: insurer): ■ homeopathy.: 135 patients; minimum of one homeopathic remedy, no psychotropic medicines: 53.46 € ■ psychiatry: 185 patients; minimum of one psychotropic medicine and no homeopathic remedy: 65.75 €	Both strategies were equally effective (Hamilton Anxiety Scale, Likert Scale, Spielberger State Trait Anxiety Inventory). The authors conclude potential cost savings with homeopathic treatment.
changes in the use of conventional medicine: ■ 29% could able to stop conventional medication, 33% reduced dosage, 32% reported 'no change' and 6% increased the medication. ■ The state of health (mean value from score) improved slightly during the observation period. 29% of overall costs were due to consultation time, 22% of overall costs were due to CAM medication.	The authors conclude a potential cost reduction with homeopathic treatment due to cutting down on expenses for conventional medication. They state that calculations are possible without conducting an RCT, e.g. as prospective data assessment. The authors emphasize how important an economic evaluation of the method is and predict that homeopathy will be increasingly accepted once its cost-effectiveness is better known.

◼ Table 12.2 (continued)

Author, year, title	Country	Method	Participant, diagnosis	
Van Haselen et al (1999) The costs of treating rheumatoid arthritis patients with complementary medicine: exploring the issue	UK	Pilot project to evaluate the costs of homeopathic treatment for rheumatic complaints (retrospective evaluation). All patients had had conventional treatment and started homeopathic treatment at the beginning of the evaluation period.	89 patients with rheumatic disorders (random sample)	
Van Wassenhoven and Ives (2004) An observational study of patients receiving homeopathic treatment	Belgium	patient interviews (retrospective) and evaluation	782 patients from 80 practices, homeopathically treated	
Wiesenauer et al (1992) Naturheilkunde als Beitrag zur Kostendämpfung	Germany	Descriptive evaluation of data of a statutory health insurer (KV Nord-Wurttemberg, second quarter of 1988): comparison of medical practitioners with additional homeopathic and/or naturopathic qualifications.		
Wemmer (1997). Gesundheitspolitik – Kostendämpfung durch Antihomotoxika bei der Behandlung grippaler Infekte	Germany	Cost comparison of daily costs with conventional and homeopathic treatment (theoretical calculation based on assessment of medicine consumption in individual cases)	influenza-like infection	

1 German medical fee schedule
2 No calculations given for time expended/costs of allopathic treatment; similar costs are assumed, as the fee schedule does not include expenses for homeopathic consultation.
3 CNAMTS-statistics (CNAMTS = Caisse Nationale d'Assurance Maladie des Travailleurs Salariés)
4 preparations such as solutions for infusion are also included
5 very sparse documentation, e.g. unclear how the comparative data for the 'area' were collected. Number of participating physicians too small too allow for reliable conclusions.
6 all consultations: NHS + out of pocket
7 first consultation based on this diagnosis; diagnosed according to DSM IV

Results	Comments
overall costs of treatment for 89 patients: £ 7632, of which: ■ £ 1681 consultation time ■ £ 1617 X-rays ■ £ 1535 medication	The authors see potential cost advantage with homeopathic therapy due to cutting down on expenses for conventional medication. The results of this first investigation need to be confirmed by further studies.
Mean consultation time: ■ 37 min (homeopathic physician) ■ 15 min (conventional physician) With 52% of patients one or several of the previously used conventional medicaments could be discontinued. The costs of the prescribed homeopathic medication were only a third of the costs for general prescriptions in Belgium. 27% of patients had simultaneous conventional treatment for their condition.	Validity of study restricted due to quality of retrospective data. The authors conclude potential cost savings by using homeopathy and request further research with prospective assessment and better instruments.
average costs/treatment Calculation was based on the regular dosage using 1995 prices in Deutschmark: ■ antitussive drugs: DM 1.39–1.47 ■ expectorants: DM 1.39 ■ antihomotoxic products: DM 0.35–0.94 ■ conventional flu medicine: DM 1.67 ■ conventional. rhinol. drugs: DM 0.32–1.37	The author concludes potential cost savings with homeopathic medicines in the treatment of influenza-like infections.

■ **Table 12.3** Homeopathy: clinical studies that assessed resource consumption as well as clinical parameters (main focus on indication selected for HTA: upper respiratory tract infections/allergies)

Author, year, title	Method	Participants
Eizayaga and Eizayaga (1996) Homeopathic treatment of bronchial asthma	retrospective investigation	62 patients, bronchial asthma
Frei (2001) Homeopathy in acute otitis media in children: treatment effect or spontaneous resolution?	treatment	230 children, otitis media
Friese (1997) The homeopathic treatment of otitis media in children – comparisons with conventional therapy	prospective, controlled, not randomized study, comparison with conventional treatment (incl. antibiotics)	131 children, otitis media
Harrison H (1999) A randomized comparison of homeopathic and standard care for the treatment of glue ear in children	not blinded, randomiszed study (pilot project); comparison with conventional treatment	32 children, otitis media
Reilly (1986) Is homeopathy a placebo response? Controlled trial of homeopathic potency, with pollen in hay fever as model	RCT, placebo-controlled	144 patients, hay fever
Taylor (2000) Randomized controlled trial of homeopathy versus placebo on perennial allergic rhinitis with overview of four trial series	RCT, placebo-controlled	50 patients, allergic rhinitis
Weber (2002) A non-randomized pilot study to compare complementary and conventional treatments to acute sinusitis	multi-centre, non-randomized, controlled study	63 patients, acute sinusitis

1 The difference was even more pronounced when the number of responders in the respective treatment group was also considered in the analysis.

185

12

Results	Comments
assessment of discontinuation of conventional drugs: corticosteroids – 13/18 patients (72.2%), theophylline – 10/14 (71.4%) and beta-adrenergic drugs – 9/31 (29%)	Despite the methodological restrictions of a retrospective evaluation , the results highlight the homeopaths' daily experience of the effectiveness of treatments and support the request for further research. They also underline the importance of choosing the right remedy, as otherwise the effect can be reduced.
The authors calculated costs based on information concerning Switzerland; treatment costs in the homeopathy group were 14% lower than those in the conventional group (antibiotics, nasal spray).	
Freedom from recurrence after 1 year was 70.7% in the homeopathy group and 56.5% in the conventional group (p not given). Five of 103 children received additional antibiotics in the homeopathically treated group, compared to with 23 out of 28 children in the conventionally treated group.	The authors conclude from the results that homeopathic treatment of otitis media offers a good and safe alternative to conventional treatment with antibiotics.
The difference between the groups with regard to antibiotic consumption and referral to a specialist consultant was were lower in the homeopathic group (no statistical significance).	
The use of antihistamines was significantly lower in the homeopathic group (average number of tablets in 2 weeks 11.2, SD: 13.5) than in the placebo group (average number of tablets in 2 weeks 19.7, SD: 18.6)[8]. No information on dosage given.	
reduction of antihistamine consumption	
While in the conventional group 32/33 patients were given antibiotics, 32/33 patients sympathomimetics and 5/33 analgesics, these drugs were not used in the homeopathic group. Here, 26/30 patients used Sinopret* in addition (only one patient in the conventional group) and 20/30 patients used inhalation (12 patients in the conventional group).	The authors conclude comparable effectiveness in both treatment groups, while pointing out that the groups were not homogeneous and therefore not fully comparable. In order to demonstrate therapeutic equivalence a patient number of 400 would be necessary.

Table 12.4 Pilot projects carried out by Statutory Health Insurers (source: German Federal Health Report)

Insurer	Permitted treatment	Inclusion criteria	Volume
Betriebskranken-kassen[2] in the districts of Essen, Oldenburg, Cologne (21 funds in total)	various CAM treatments[3]	chronically ill patients; all conventional treatment options exhausted	1200 patients for Essen and Cologne. Own medical fee schedule; approx. DM 16.8 m for treatment (incl. dentist costs and external services) through the entire test period (1994–2001); evaluative research DM 1.2 m.
BV IKK, IKK Saxony, IKK Saxony-Anhalt, IKK Baden-Württemberg	acupuncture, homeopathy	all insurance members	5000 patients DM 60/session (approx. DM 3.4 m. treatment costs up to 08/2000; evaluative research ca. DM 800,000
BKK LV NRW[4], KV Westfalen Lippe[5]	seven naturopathic therapies	chronically, severely ill insured patients; all conventional treatment options exhausted	918 patients
IKK Hamburg	homeopathy, anthroposophic medicine	lumbar spine syndrome, coxarthrosis, gonarthrosis, sleeping disorders, depressive syndrome, migraine, allergic rhinitis, bronchial asthma, neurodermatitis, chronic sinusitis, chronic tonsillitis	ca. 1000 patients scheduled in alternative treatment group
BKK Post[13]	acupuncture, homeopathy	head and back pain, atopic disorders	scheduled: 15,000 patients DM 70/patient and session + DM 534,000 for evaluative research (3 years)
LV BKK, KV Bayern, BKK BMW, BKK Siemens, BKK Allianz	various CAM treatments[2]	chronic headache, back pain, neurodermatitis	376 patients, physicians compensation based on flat rate of DM 600 for the entire observation period, GOÄ/EBM[3] items; evaluative research DM 800,000 (in total)
Techniker-krankenkasse[4]	acupuncture	allergic rhinitis, allergic asthma, lumbar spine syndrome, cervical spine syndrome, headaches, dysmenorrhoea	scheduled: 30,000 patients/year, DM 30 m/year, estimated.: 70 DM/session, 10% of which paid by patient

▣ Table 12.4 (continued)

Insurer	Permitted treatment	Inclusion criteria	Volume
AOK[5], IKK, BKK (some exceptions), Knappschaft[6]; Landwirtschaftliche Krankenkassen[7], Seekasse[8]	acupuncture with sham acupuncture (as specified by the German federal commission of physicians: *Bundesausschuss Ärzte*)	chronic tension headache, migraine, chronic lumbar spine complaints, coxarthrosis, chronicity >6 months	scheduled: cohort with 120,000 AOK and 80,000 BKK/IKKn patients per year and DM 50/session; DM 8 m for evaluative research; randomisation: 4000 patients DM 15 m for evaluative research
all substitute funds (apart from Technikerkrankenkasse)	acupuncture with sham acupuncture (as specified by Bundesausschuss Ärzte)	chronic tension headache, migraine, chronic lumbar spine syndrome, chronic joint pain with osteoarthrosis, chronicity >6 months	scheduled: more than 100,000 patients at 50 DM/session + DM 10 for A-diploma holders or DM 20 for B-diploma holders; scheduled: DM 1,.3 m for treatment within randomisation study; evaluative research DM 4.4 m

1 Gesundheitsberichterstattung des Bundes, Heft 9 *Inanspruchnahme alternativer Methoden in der Medizin*, Marstedt and Moebus 2001
2 BKK – statutory health insurer in Germany
3 anamnesis decoder, Lüscher Test, regulation thermography, electro-acupuncture, measuring of oral electric current (diagnosis) acupuncture, neural therapy, homeopathy, colon-hydrotherapy, haematogenous oxidation therapy, oxygen therapies (with exceptions), physiotherapy, reflexology, vitamins and minerals, isotherapy and symbiotic control/ microbiological therapy (treatment)
4 BKK LV NRW: Betriebskrankenkasse Landesverband Nordrhein Westfalen
5 KV: Kassenärztliche Vereinigung (Association of statutory health insurance physicians)
6 post offices sickness insurance fund
7 classical naturopathic therapies (nutrition and movement therapy/massage, hydro-/thermotherapy, lifestyle/regulative therapy, phytotherapy), acupuncture (body, ear), neural therapy, physiotherapy
8 GOÄ/EBM: Gebührenordnung für Ärzte/ Einheitlicher Bewertungsmaßstab Ärzte (medical fee schedule for physicians/ standard fee scale physicians)
9 Technicians' sickness insurance fund
10 AOK: Allgemeine Ortskrankenkasse (Local health insurance provider in Germany)
11 miners' sickness insurance fund
12 agricultural sickness insurance fund
13 seamen's sickness insurance fund

The restrictions mentioned are known and are being discussed in the literature. Friedman et al. (1997) has already suggested that different CAM definitions lead to different cost-calculation results. The authors criticize that behavioural therapies which are proven to contribute to cost savings are often not included in the established CAM definitions. They conclude that cost savings are underestimated if such methods are not included in an analysis.

In an overview on CAM, Lewith (2000) also arrives at the conclusion that not sufficient data are not yet available yet to reliably evaluate the cost- effectiveness of CAM. There are only individual studies on homeopathy (van Haselen 2000) and acupuncture (Stewart et al. 2001), both of which both corroborate the cost- effectiveness of the respective approach. The largest survey which was carried out by a French health insurer also suggests lower costs for homeopathy (Chaufferin 2000, Taieb and Myon 2003, Trichard et al. 2003). Due to the increase in CAM use, Lewith (2000) asks calls for adequate studies to be carried out to establish cost- effectiveness.

For Switzerland only one study is available on the cost-effectiveness of CAM (Sommer et al. 1999), in which the authors infer an additive usage of CAM. Publication of the study and its conclusions have has given rise to widespread discussion (Heusser 1999, Kienle and Kiene 1999, Studer 1999). Points of criticism were mostly structural and question the conclusions drawn by the authors from the collected data. The inference of additive usage in particular cannot be derived from the data available. The most important aspects are, in brief:

- The study period of 2 years was shorter than planned and therefore too short to assess sustained improvement. Many of the insured only took advantage of the benefits only at the end of the project.
- In 1993, the Swiss insurance provider *Helvetia* introduced the additional insurance of up to CHF SFR 500 also for the control group, which means that the comparison with insurance providers or insurance holders with and without additional insurance is not valid.
- Only 1.1% of insurance-holders took advantage of the offer.
- Lack of comparability of groups: in the experimental group the percentage of patients with high health-care costs in 1991was higher in the experimental group than in the control groups.
- The state of health was only assessed for only 10 ten patients; therefore no conclusions are possible.
- Assessing the state of health in telephone interviews doses not meet the criteria for the scientific application of questionnaire SF-36.

German pilot projects indicate sustained effectiveness for CAM therapies: Two pilot projects showed a definite and sustained decrease in sick- leave days before and after treatment begin from 32 before to 23 or 24 days in the second observation year. The data suggest at least the potential for indirect cost savings. Data concerning direct costs cannot be drawn from the pilot projects.

Cost- effectiveness studies on individual complementary medical treatments clearly indicate possible savings. Various investigations are available for homeopathy and physical therapies.

12.12.3   Homeopathy

The economic aspects of homeopathy have been increasingly considered in recent years. Apart from studies and other surveys, comments and summaries on the subject are published more and more frequently in various journals:

Schüppel et al. (2003) conclude from a review of the published data that, with the current costs of pharmaceutical products, the use of homeopathy has the potential to lower pharmaceutical spending. Further studies are needed to evaluate whether the costs per case will remain lower over a longer period of time than those of conventional treatment.

In the meantime, some of the authors have conducted a more specific systematic review with cost minimalization analysis (Maxion-Bergemann et al. "Cost minimalization analysis of homeopathy and conventional medicine based on a systematic literature review", submitted). They conclude: 'Available data suggest potential cost savings due to the use of homeopathy. Further well-designed studies and analyses of existing databases for homeopathy are encouraged in order to support informed decisions in European health-care systems.'

12.13   References

Alvarez JLA (2005) Cuba's public health system before and after the introduction of homeopathy, results of a study. Available at: www.liga2005.de

Andrews GJ, Peter E, Hammond R (2003) Receiving money for medicine: some tensions and resolutions for community-based private complementary therapists. Health Soc Care Commun 1:155–167

Astin JA, Marie A, Pelletier KR, Hansen E, Haskell WL (1998) A review of the incorporation of complementary and alternative medicine by mainstream physicians. Arch Intern Med 158:2303–2310

Becker-Witt C, Lüdtke R, Willich SN (2003) Patienten in der homöopathischen Praxis. In: Albrecht H, Frühwald M, (eds) Jahrbuch 9, Karl und Veronika Carstens-Stiftung. KVC Verlag, Essen pp 3–15

Bleul G (1997) Kostenvergleich Homöopathie/konventionelle Medizin am Beispiel zweier Fälle von akutem Tinnitus. Allgem homöopatische Zeitung 242:190–198

Bolis M (2003) Consumo nazionale della medicina omeopathica: analisi empirica sulla base dell'Indagine sulla salute in Svizzera. Lavoro di diploma, Scuola Universitaria Professionale della Svizzera Italiana (SUSPI), Manno, Switzerland (Publikation auch im Rahmen des Newsletter PEK)

Bradford TL (1984) The logic of figures: or comparative results of homeopathic and other treatments (1900). Homeopathic Educational Services, Berkeley, CA

Breu E (1999) Kommentar zur Nationalfondsstudie "Komplementärmedizin in der Grundversicherung. Verteuert sie die Gesundheitskosten? svha/ssmh-bulletin 4:6–7

Buchbinder R, Gingold M, Hall S, Cohen M (2002) Non-prescription complementary treatments used by rheumatoid arthritis patients attending a community-based rheumatology practice. Intern Med J 32:208–214

Bundesamt für Statistik (ed) (2003) StatSanté. Resultate zu den Gesundheitsstatistiken in der Schweiz. Gesundheitskosten in der Schweiz: Entwicklung von 1960 bis 2000. Neuchatel, available at: http://www.bfs.admin.ch/bfs/portal/de/index/themen/gesundheit/uebersicht/blank/publikationen.Document.26245.pdf

Buxton M (2000) Assessing the cost-effectiveness of homeopathic medicines: are the problems different from other health technologies? Br Homeopathic J 89:20–22

Chaufferin G (2000) Improving the evaluation of homeopathy: economic considerations and impact on health. Br Homeopathic J 89:27–30

Christen P, Erlach A, Etter G, Geissbühler H, Roth R, Siles C, Walser T, Wegmüller A (2000) "Drop-out"-PatientInnen in der Homöopathie: eine Befragung zur Zufriedenheit in der homöopathischen Behandlung. svha/ssmh bulletin 5:4–5. available at: http://www.homeodoctor.ch/dropout.htm

Conrad DA, Maynard C, Cheadle A, Ramsey S, Marcus-Smith M, Kirz H, Madden CA, Martin D, Perrin EB, Wickizer T, Zierler B, Ross A, Noren J, Liang S-Y (1998) Primary care physician compensation method in medical groups: does it influence the use and cost of health services for enrollees in managed CAM organizations? JAMA 279: 853–858

De Lange de Klerk ESM, Blommers J, Kruik DJ, Bezemer PD, Feenstra L (1994) Effect of homeopathic medicines on daily burden of symptoms in children with recurrent upper respiratory tract infections. BMJ 309:1329–1332

Dixon A, Riesberg A, Weinbrenner S, Saka O, Le Grand J, Busse R (2003) Complementary and alternative medicine in the UK and Germany – research and evidence on supply and demand. Anglo-German Foundation for the Study of Industrial Society/Deutsch-Britische Stiftung für das Studium der Industriegesellschaft. London Berlin. available at: http://www.mig.tu-berlin.de/files/2003.publications/2003.dickson_CAM.report.2003.pdf

Drähne A (1991) Kostenersparnis durch homöopathische Therapie. In: Dokumentation der besonderen Therapierichtungen und natürlichen Heilweisen in Europa. VGM Essen

Egede LE, Ye X, Zheng D, Silverstein MD (2002) The prevalence and pattern of complementary and alternative medicine use in individuals with diabetes. Diabetes Care 25:324–329

Eisebitt R 1999) Methodik gesundheitsökonomischer Studien in der Komplementärmedizin unter besonderer Berücksichtigung der Homöopathie. HomInt R&D Newslett (1:4–10

Eisenberg DM, Davis RB, Ettner SL, Appel S, Wilkey S, Van Rompay M, Kessler RC (1998) Trends in alternative medicine use in the United States, 1990–1997: results of a follow-up national survey. JAMA 280:1569–1575

Eisenberg DM, Kessler RC, Foster C, Norlock FE, Calkins DR, Delbanco TL (1993) Unconventional medicine in the United States: prevalence, costs and patterns of use. N Engl J Med 328:246–252

Eizayaga FX, Eizayaga J (1996) Homeopathic treatment of bronchial asthma. Retrospective study of 62 cases. Br Homeopathic J 85:28–33

Ernst E, White A (2000) The BBC survey of complementary medicine use in the UK. Complement Ther Med 8:32–36

Fairfield KM, Eisenberg DM, Davis RB, Libman H, Phillips RS (1998) Patterns of use, expenditures, and perceived efficacy of complementary and alternative therapies in HIV-infected patients. Arch Intern Med 158:2257–2264

Feldhaus HW (1993) Cost-effectiveness of homeopathic treatment in a dental practice. Br Homeopathic J 82:22–28

Frei H, Thurneysen A (2001) Homeopathy in acute otitis media in children: treatment effect or spontaneous resolution? Br Homeopathic J 90:180–182

Frenkel M, Hermoni D (2002) Effects of homeopathic intervention on medication consumption in atopic and allergic disorders. Altern Ther Health Med 8:76–79

Friedman R, Sedler M, Myers P, Benson H (1997) Behavioral medicine, complementary medicine and integrated care. Economic implications. Prim Care 24:949–962

Friese K-H, Kruse S, Lüdtke R, Moeller H (1997) The homeopathic treatment of otitis media in children – comparisons with conventional therapy. Int J Clin Pharmacol Ther 35:296–301

Furler MD, Einarson TR, Walmsley S, Millson M, Bandayan R (2003) Use of complementary and alternative medicine by HIV-infected outpatients in Ontario, Canada. AIDS Pat Care STDs 17:155–168

Gerhard I, Reimers G, Keller C, Schmück M (1993) Vergleich homöopathischer Einzelmittel mit konventioneller Hormontherapie. Therapeutikon 7:309–315

Gmür R (2003) Fallkosten in der Psychotherapie. Schweiz Arztezeitung 84:638–640

Güthlin C, Lange O, Walach H (2004) Measuring the effects of acupuncture and homeopathy in general practice: an uncontrolled prospective documentation approach. BMC Public Health 4(6)

Güthlin C, Walach H (2001) Prospektive Dokumentationsstudie in der niedergelassenen Praxis – ein Erprobungsverfahren zur Akupunktur und Homöopathie. Erfahrungsheilkunde 50:186–194

Haidvogl M, Riley DS, Heger M (2001) Effectiveness and costs of homeopathy compared to conventional medicine in the outpatient care setting. In: The Royal London Homeopathic Hospital (ed) Improving the success of homeopathy. 3:71–72

Harrison H, Fixsen A, Vickers A (1999) A randomized comparison of homeopathic and standard care for the treatment of glue ear in children. Complement Ther Med 7:132–135

Heger M, Riley DS, Haidvogl M (2000) International integrative primary care outcomes study (IIPCOS-2): an international research project of homeopathy in primary care. Br Homeopathic J 89:10–13

Heger M, Riley DS, Haidvogl M, Gordon D, Herrick N, Wolscher U, Thurneysen A (2001) IIPCOS – Ein internationales Projekt zur Untersuchung der Effektivität der Homöopathie in der ärztlichen Primärversorgung. HomInt R&D Newslett 2:3–19

Heusser P (1999) Komplementärmedizin in der Grundversicherung: verteuert sie die Gesundheitskosten? Schweiz Z GanzheitsMed 11:4–9

Hills D, Welford R (1998) Complementary therapy in general practice, an evaluation of the Glastonbury Health Centre Complementary Medicine Service. available at: http://www.integratedhealth.org.uk/report.html

Junker J, Oberwittler C, Jackson D, Berger K (2004) Utilization and perceived effectiveness of complementary and alternative medicine in patients with dystonia. Mov Disord 19:158–161

Keil K (2001) Clinical outcomes of a diagnostic and treatment protocol in allergy/sensitivity patients. Altern Med Rev 6:188–202

Kienle GS, Kiene H (1999) Können aus der Studie „Komplementärmedizin in der Krankenversicherung" wissenschaftlich tragfähige Schlüsse gezogen werden? Forschende Komplementärmedizin 6:262–270

Lewith GT (2000) A provider's perspective: current issues in providing and funding complementary medical care. Forschende Komplementärmedizin und Klassische Naturheilkunde 7:242–246

MacLennan AH, Wilson DH, Taylor AW (1996) Prevalence and costs of alternative medicine in Australia. Lancet 347:569–573

Marstedt G, Moebus S (2002) Gesundheitsberichterstattung des Bundes Heft 9: Inanspruchnahme alternativer Methoden in der Medizin. Verlag Robert Koch Institut, Berlin

Marx HH (1997) The dilemma of effectiveness and economic value of alternative medicine. [in German]. Gesundheitswesen 59:297–301

Moebus S, Hirche H, Ose C, Jöckel KH (1998) Naturmedizin und Therapiekosten: erste Ergebnisse einer Machbarkeitsstudie. Naturamed 13:16–23

Müller C (2000) Neues vom Hausarztsystem EGK-SVHA. svha/ssmh bulletin 5:17

Patterson RE, Neuhouser ML, Hedderson MM, Schwartz SM, Standish LJ, Bowen DJ, Marshall LM (2002) Types of alternative medicine used by patients with breast, colon, or prostate cancer: predictors, motives, and costs. J Altern Complement Med 8:477–485

Pelletier KR, Astin JA (2002) Integration and reimbursement of complementary and alternative medicine by managed care and insurance providers: 2000 update and cohort analysis. Altern Ther Health Med 8:38–39, 42, 44

Ramsey SD, Spencer AC, Topolski TD, Belza B, Patrick DL (2001) Use of alternative therapies by older adults with osteoarthritis. Arthritis Care Res 45:222–227

Rees RW, Feigel I, Vickers A, Zollman C, McGurk R, Smith C (2000) Prevalence of complementary therapy use by women with breast cancer: a population-based survey. Eur J Cancer 36:1359–1364

Reilly DT, McSharry C, Taylor MA, Aitchison T (1986) Is homeopathy a placebo response? Controlled trial of homeopathic potency with pollen in hay fever as model. Lancet 2:881–886

Riley D, Fisher M SB, Haidvogl M, Heger M (2001) Homeopathy and conventional medicine: an outcomes study comparing effectiveness in a primary care setting. J Altern Complement Med 7:149–159

Schafer T, Riehle A, Wichmann HE, Ring J (2002) Alternative medicine in allergies – prevalence, patterns of use, and costs. Allergy 57:694–700

Schlüren E (1984) Vergleich der Arzneimittelkosten bei homöopathischer und allopathisch-schulmedizinischer Behandlung. Vergleich der Arzneimittelkosten. Allgem Homöopathische Zeitung 229:160–161

Schmidt JM (2001) Taschenatlas Homöopathie in Wort und Bild. Haug, Heidelberg

Schüppel R (2003) Kosten und Nutzen der Homöopathie – ein echtes Schnäppchen? Hausarzt 19:64

Shenfield G, Lim E, Allen H (2002) Survey of the use of complementary medicines and therapies in children with asthma. J Paediatr Child Health 38:252–257

Slade K, Chohan BP, Barker PJ (2004) Evaluation of a GP practice-based homeopathy service. Homeopathy 93:67–70

Sommer JH, Burgi M (1999) A randomized experiment of the effects of including alternative medicine in the mandatory benefit package of health insurance funds in Switzerland. Complement Ther Med 7:54–61

Sommer JH (1999) Gesundheitsökonomische Analyse der Wirkungen des Angebots komplementärmedizinischer Leistungen der Krankenkassen. Forschende Komplementärmedizin 6:7–9

Sommer JH, Burgi M, Theiss R (1999) Inclusion of complementary medicine increases health costs. Focus Altern Complement Ther 4:183–184

Stewart D, Weeks J, Bent S (2001) Utilization, patient satisfaction, and cost implications of acupuncture, massage, and naturopathic medicine offered as covered health benefits: a comparison of two delivery models. Altern Ther Health Med 7:66–70

Studer HP (1999) Natürliches Heilen spart Kosten und fördert die Gesundheit. Schweizer Verband für natürliches Heilen, Bern

Studer HP, Busato A: Ist ärztliche Komplementärmedizin wirtschaftlich? SchweizÄrzteZeitung 2010;91(18):707–721

Studer HP, Busato A: Development of Costs for Complementary Medicine after Provisional Inclusion into the Swiss Basic Health Insurance. Forsch Komplementmed 2011;18:15–23

Swayne J (1992) The cost and effectiveness of homeopathy. Br Homeopathic J 81:148–150

Taieb C, Myon E (2003) The economic impact of homeopathic management: the French example. Value Health 6:373

Taylor MA, Reilly D, Llewellyn-Jones RH, McSharry C, Aitchison TC (2000) Randomized controlled trial of homeopathy versus placebo in perennial allergic rhinitis with overview of four trial series. BMJ 321:471–476

Thomas KJ, Nicholl JP, Coleman P (2001) Use and expenditure on complementary medicine in England: a population-based survey. Complement Ther Med 9:2–11

Trichard M, Chaufferin G, Nicoloyannis N (2003) Pharmacoeconomic comparison between two drug strategies of treatment of anxiety disorders: homeopathy and psychotropics (ISPOR Poster PMH23). Value Health 6:350–351

Van Haselen R (2000) The economic evaluation of complementary medicine: a staged approach at the Royal London Homeopathic Hospital. Br Homeopathic J 89 [Suppl 1]:S23–26

Van Haselen R, Fisher P (1999) Attitudes to evidence on complementary medicine: the perspective of British healthcare purchasers. Complement Ther Med 7:136–141

Van Haselen RA, Graves N, Dahiha S (1999) The costs of treating rheumatoid arthritis patients with complementary medicine: Exploring the issue. Complement Ther Med 7:217–221

van Wassenhoven M, Ives G A(2004) n observational study of patients receiving homeopathic treatment. Homeopathy 93:3–11

Vickers AJ (1994) Complementary therapies on the NHS: The NAHAT survey. Complementary Therapies in Medicine 2:48–50

Von Gruenigen VE, White LJ, Kirven MS, Showalter AL, Hopkins MP, Jenison EL (2001) A comparison of complementary and alternative medicine use by gynecology and gynecologic oncology patients. Int J Gynecol Cancer 11:205–209

Walach H, Schüller S, Heinrich S, Eßer P (1997) The test phase of the Innungskrankenkassen on acupuncture and homeopathy. Forschende Komplementärmedizin 4:121

Weber U, Lüdtke R., Friese K.H., Fischer I, Moeller H (2002) A non-randomized pilot study to compare complementary and conventional treatments of acute sinusitis. Forschende Komplementärmedizin 9:99–104

Wemmer U (1997) Gesundheitspolitik – Kostendämpfung durch Antihomotoxika bei der Behandlung Grippaler Infekte. Biol Med 5:218–222

White A, Slade P, Hunt C, Hart A, Ernst E (2003) Individualized homeopathy as an adjunct in the treatment of childhood asthma: a randomized placebo-controlled trial. Thorax 58:317–321

White AR, Resch KL, Ernst E (1996) Methods of economic evaluation in complementary medicine. Forschende Komplementärmedizin 3:196–203

Wiesenauer M, Groh P, Häußler S (1992) Naturheilkunde als Beitrag zur Kostendämpfung. Fortschr Med 110:31–38

12

Full discussion
of the HTA results

Gudrun Bornhöft, Klaus v. Ammon, Marco Righetti,
André Thuneysen and Peter F. Matthiessen

It was the task of the present HTA to evaluate, within the PEK[1] context, the efficacy, appropriateness (in terms of demand and safety) and economy of homeopathy. For this purpose the situation in Switzerland had to be assessed and reflected as realistically as possible.

The literature was selected from internet accessible data bases on the one hand and via expert contacts and scanning of bibliographical reference lists on the other. Just searching online would not have been sufficient to supply a representative overview of homeopathic research. The results were too broad: the search terms 'systematic review' and 'meta-analysis' produced more than 300 hits in our specially generated homeopathy database. The revision of titles and abstracts left us with only 22 'genuine reviews'. The search was also not comprehensive enough and we had to find more reviews, clinical trials and above all studies on the use, safety and cost effectiveness of homeopathy through expert contacts and scanning of bibliographical references. Our research for the domain Upper Respiratory Tract Infection/ Allergy (URTI/A studies) showed that only a limited number of studies could be found despite an extensive web search in the indexed literature and authors' reference lists and that the search in homeopathic practices supplied numerous other studies. One can assume that a systematic search in countries where homeopathy is wide-spread (e.g. Latin America, India) would produce far more URTI/A studies.

The problem could be due to the still lingering scepticism of 'established' journals towards CAM and homeopathy in particular, but the indexing of CAM articles also still seems to be rudimentary and inconsistent so that not all articles of a database can be located.

With its special characteristics homeopathy does not seem to be compatible with the current (mechanistic-molecular) paradigmatic model, especially the use of non-substantial high potencies. Its most prominent traits are the choice of treatment based on the similarity principle, i.e. the substance that causes the same symptoms in the healthy person as those displayed by the patient, the meticulous observation of all manifesting symptoms and individual signs in the patient with a view to the choice of remedy and the use of potentized substances that are diluted in a special process.

Naturopathy uses Arnica to heal wounds because it has been proven to be effective, but does not consider the fact that it can evoke similar muscle and pain symptoms in a healthy person.

Medicines that are potentized to $\geq$ D24 and $\geq$ C12 are far more controversial as there is usually no molecule of the active agent left in the dilutions.

The progress achieved in physics means that subatomic models are available to explain the action of highly potentized homeopathic medicines (imprint theory, coherence of cellular and subcellular energy analogous to the coherence of laser light etc.), but it has not been possible so far to prove that they apply to homeopathy.

Fundamental research mainly focuses on the mode of action of highly potentized substances in order to explain their paradigm-opposing effectiveness in a clear and comprehensible manner and can be summarized as follows:

Many high quality studies of preclinical fundamental research support the homeopathic view that even highly potentized medicines are able to induce specific effects in living organisms. Homeopathic medicines moreover appear to have a regulatory, i.e. balancing or normalizing, effect and possess a specific physical structure. Fundamental preclinical research is for reasons of non-transferability not able to evaluate the other basic tenets of homeopathy (simile rule and drug proving on the healthy person).

---

1   Programm Evaluation Komplementärmedizin

Another special aspect of homeopathy is phenomenological (and interactional) in nature and lies in the fact that it does not strive to quickly summarize, abstract and classify the symptoms into a diagnosis (i.e. attribute them to a virtual disease entity) to find the right medication but focuses on the entirety of individual, idiosyncratic and conspicuous symptoms and signs of the patient, takes them seriously, although conventional medicine often ridicules or neglects phenomena such as sensitivity to weather conditions, dreams, biorhythmic symptoms, food preferences and aversions or psychological characteristics. Homeopathy sees these individual symptoms as outer expressions (*gestalt*) of an inner process that cannot be observed (disease, 'regulatory disturbance', 'disturbance of the vital force' – *Verstimmung der Lebenskraft* – according to Hahnemann). Unlike with conventional history taking, patients feel they are perceived without being devaluated which can considerably affect their ability to release physical and mental blockages and activate their own regulatory powers. Linde (1998) even assumes that this effect – to which both verum and control group are equally 'exposed' – can be so strong within the context of an RCT that the actual effect of the homeopathic medication is masked and the difference between verum and placebo group is reduced to non-significance. It would therefore make more sense to examine the 'system of homeopathic treatment' which includes factors such as the symptom-based modification of the homeopathic substance instead of testing a particular 'freely prepared' active agent in the interest of academic correctness.

For this reason we decided to base our evaluation not only on the usual randomized controlled trials (RCTs), but to include other study designs as well. The reservations concerning a purely RCT based literature analysis do not only apply to homeopathy but also – if to a lesser degree – to other fields of clinical research, especially if more complex interventions are involved. (Cf. Chapter 5)

They are here again briefly summarized:

1. The absence of a positive or any RCT result is no proof of ineffectiveness ('absence of evidence is not evidence of absence', Altman & Bland 1995); there is a danger that effective therapies are eliminated because there is no RCT proof of their efficacy.

2. A negative RCT result is also not valid proof of ineffectiveness because many factors can be involved in causing false-negative RCT results. Vice versa, the absence of many factors that are excluded by the RCT design can be responsible for false negative results, such as a disturbed doctor-patient relationship, non-compliance, drop-outs (with ITT analysis), complementary and compensatory therapy, but also mega-studies with their – necessarily – simplified study-design.

3. Individualized medical care is more and more replaced by standardized treatment methods to ensure comparability and reproducibility of study outcomes.

4. Trial results can be significantly positive even though only a small percentage of patients experiences genuine benefit from the trial. This applies particularly to trials with large, but generally heterogeneous, patient collectives. The results do not allow for conclusions as to which patients (or sub-groups) benefited and which did not benefit (or sustained damage from the treatment). In preventive medicine, a 'number needed to treat' (NNT) of 100 to 200 subjects is still considered sensible! One must ask how many people can be expected to use a medication that is of no benefit to them in order to help one individual in the group? Study results can, on the other hand, come out negative although a percentage of the patients drew definite benefit from the treatment. With most trials the statistical significance is not enough to discriminate even major differences in the subgroups (cf. Niroomand 2004).

5. Reproducibility is surprisingly low even with 'hard' RCTs (rigorous inclusion criteria, end-points with minimal subjectivity). There are also ethical concerns which prohibit repetition of RCTs with a positive outcome (in favour of the test intervention) because the patients in the control group would be denied a treatment that is known to be effective.

6. This is not the only ethical reason why there needs to be genuine openness ('equipoise') at the beginning of a randomized trial, i.e. neither physician nor patient have a preference regarding a particular treatment. The fact that a patient has given his or her 'informed con-sent' does not avoid the problem either since the responsibility cannot simply be placed on the patient, certainly not according to the Declaration of the World Medical Association: 'The responsibility for the human subject must always rest with a medically qualified person and never rest on the subject of the research, even though the subject has given consent.' (Quoted from Kienle et al. 2006b) Equipoise, in fact, only applies to the classical usage of RCTs i.e. the testing of new medicines on which the terms 'preclinical' and 'clinical research' and 'phase I, II, III and IV trials' is based. It is doubtful whether RCTs are suitable for the evaluation of complex therapeutic procedures or of entire therapy systems that have been part of the day-to-day primary health care provision for decades.

7. In view of the ethical problems mentioned it appears doubtful whether the authorities have the right to insist on randomized trials, i.e. evidence of inferior treatment and discrimination of control group patients, as a basis for decisions concerning health service reimbursement. To quote Gerhard Kienle: 'If authorities, beyond the ethically and legally demanded duty of self-sacrifice, make *experiments on humans* a precondition for the availability of certain medicines to the physician, necessary to fulfil his treatment obligation, then they are exerting a compul-sion through which the study participant will become the means to an end. This act falls within Kant's definition of immorality.' (Kienle 1974, p. 23, quoted from Kienle et al. 2006b).

8. 'Recently the discussion for and against mammography screening exemplified how different professional evidence-based reviews of identical clinical studies could nevertheless arrive at different conclusions and even opposing recommendations on treatment' (cf. Dickersin 2003, quoted from Kienle et al. 2006b). Not only the RCT results but also the results obtained from systematic reviews of RCTs can show considerable divergence.

9. The thematic orientation of RCTs is often not relevant to problems of health care or the needs of patients, but driven by subjective interests (career, sponsors). Due to the enormous costs involved clinical research has become the domain of the pharmaceutical industry and is primarily governed by licensing and marketing interests. The generation of evidence for treatments that promise success but not financial profit or for non-pharmacological thera-pies is therefore considered dispensable.

Compared to other complementary medical methods such as phytotherapy or traditional Chinese medicine, whose basic effectiveness is hardly put into doubt by conventional medicine, the crucial point of discussion with homeopathy is the proof of effectiveness. We therefore consider it in more detail (cf. also the research by Knipschild 1989 and Knipschild & Leffers 1990, quoted from Kleijnen et al. 1991: 'The way in which the belief of people changes after the presentation of empirical evidence depends on their prior beliefs and on the quality of the evi-dence'. Kleijnen et al. continue: 'Critical people who did not believe in the efficacy of homeopa-thy before reading the evidence presented here probably will still not be convinced; people who were more ambivalent in advance will perhaps have a more optimistic view now, whereas people who already believed in the efficacy of homeopathy might at this moment be almost certain that homeopathy works').

Apart from the selection of studies the evaluation of study results plays a major part, but the question of how do deal with inconsistent study results (according to Glanville & Sowden 2001) needs to be clarified on the one hand and on the other hand the question of the qualitative evaluation or the assessment of a low, moderate or high risk of bias (Alderson et al. 2004).

- **Dealing with differing study results**

The numerous reviews that exist now on homeopathy often evaluate (overtly or covertly) the 'vote count', i.e. the number of positive and negative study results are added up and the sum total is presented as the final result: a method that we did not use in the present HTA.[2] Positive results were instead examined for risk of bias and their plausibility and an effectiveness evaluation was established on the basis of content.

- **Establishing the risk of bias:**

It has to be established in the individual case (of the individual study), differentiated according to method and content, whether the result of the positive studies is 'genuine' or whether it is biased by factors that are not related to the treatment.[3] In scientific evaluation three criteria are usually observed so that the risk of unintended bias can be assessed (conscious falsification cannot usually be recognized without knowledge of the raw data): randomization, blinding and analysis according to the intention to treat (ITT) method, where randomization is considered most important as it is meant to guarantee the equal distribution of unknown influences.[4]

Insufficient blinding involves a risk of bias in both directions: thinking that they have been given the verum, patients might give obsequious answers or there can be unconscious manipulation on the part of the evaluator in favour of the desired result which could all in all lead to false positive (or, if the evaluator 'does not like' homeopathy, to false negative) results. There is, on the other hand, greater likelihood that patients who know they do not receive the verum, use other (effective) treatment which would lead to false negative results compared to the test intervention. With homeopathy there is little danger of the test medication being 'deblinded' due to appearance, taste, smell or other reactions, which is why the authors adopted the evaluation of this criterion, if it was at all specially listed.

ITT analysis controls for attrition bias towards false positive results through unfavourable categorisation of values which are missing for the experimental treatment: all patients are evaluated on the basis of their original group affiliation irrespective of whether they completed the study or not – either with the last value carried forward (LVCF) or, in the case of dichotomous treatment evaluations, as 'treatment failures'. This method was favoured in recent years in response to the per protocol evaluation which was often criticized for omitting unfavourable results which then did not need to figure in the calculation. The reviews we evaluated also included studies from a time when ITT analyses were not so wide spread; also not all authors mentioned or extracted the kind of analysis used. Information on the number of drop outs or

---

2   It is like drawing the conclusion, after observing 2 black swans and 5 white swans, that there are no black swans, as 2-5=-3. This happens in a simple vote count or in other statistical additive procedures without thematic differentiation.

3   To stay with the picture: whether the swan is 'genuinely' black or painted or whether it seems black due to light conditions or other confounding or bias factors.

4   This is however 1) not necessarily the case, as is shown by baseline comparisons of 'well' randomized groups and 2) not to be statistically expected which is why one aims for baseline adjustment of the relevant parameters.

lost to follow-ups was usually given. In our evaluation we adhered to the customary method of assuming attrition bias with a drop-out rate $\geq 10\%$.

Even if in theory one significant study with low risk of bias is sufficient to prove the fundamental effectiveness of homeopathy, it is neither academically satisfactory to not clarify why others do not show a positive result, nor does it sufficiently reflect the real world situation, where one quite rightly asks for the frequency with which positive effects can be expected in medical healthcare. The study situation is favourable for homeopathy as there are significant positive results for various areas (e.g. overview by Mathie, 2003). These results are, however, not always consistent which led Linde (1997) to qualify their conclusion of effectiveness because no definite evidence was found in RCTs for the effectiveness of homeopathic medicines with one symptom picture. It was stated in 1998 (Linde & Melchart 1998) that if homeopathy was indeed as effective as the homeopaths claimed, there would have to be clearer proof than there had been so far. (N.B.: the importance of external validity and model validity is not considered in this argument).

If homeopathy is highly likely to be effective but this cannot be consistently proven in clinical trials, the question arises: what conditions are needed for homeopathy to show its effectiveness and to realize its potential and what conditions threaten to obscure this?[5]

Relevant contextual factors can be found through the evaluation of the external validity, e.g. the representativeness of the selected population or the question whether the chosen study design, the examination method applied, is able to answer the research question with sufficient validity also for other settings (cf. also Wein 2002 with additional model validity differentiation).

With homeopathy such context factors would be:

- Intervention: were parameters assessed that are relevant to the evaluation of the external validity (such as individualized history taking, therapy and observation of response yes/no)?
- Population: were other relevant parameters assessed apart from the indication, such as recruitment of patients etc.?
- Performance: Was information retrieved regarding the qualification of treating physicians?
- Outcome: is there evidence that differentiation was made between clinical parameters, surrogate parameters and quality of life?
- Result: Was the clinical relevance of effects taken into account?
- Safety: Were adverse events registered (and evaluated in a way that is adequate for homeopathy: initial aggravation, order of symptoms according to Hering's rule of cure?
- Follow-up: Was the length of follow-up registered and adequately evaluated for the illness? From the homeopathic point of view, too short observation periods with chronic disease and the absence of individual progress observation and treatment with RCTs are probably the factors that most severely confound external validity.

Further relevant context factors which are not yet systematically assessed or elude assessment include the organism's susceptibility to the homeopathic medicine, the homeopathic physician's expertise, the physician's certainty that he is applying the right medicine, the patient's confidence in physician and treatment, the patient's individual regulatory capacity and many more. It is

---

5   To come back to the swans: if it was known that black swans thrived particularly well in undeveloped old river arms, it would not come as a surprise if one could find and study them less in zoos, despite the fact that they could be more easily observed and analyzed there as there would be fewer confounding or bias factors.

possible that this list conceals the 'moderating factors' which must exist according to Walach (1997) (as the study results render accidentally positive results of homeopathy unlikely) but which have not yet been assessed, so that he seems more or less forced to describe the homeopathic effect as unspecific.

None of the reviews examined provided sufficient information on the factors listed above and, if they had been tentatively assessed, they were not included in the qualitative evaluation. A differentiated evaluation of the external validity of reviews was therefore hardly possible and it was mostly not sufficiently considered in the clinical studies.

From what has been described we assume a) that the purely numerical summation of positive and negative results is not adequate and we therefore did not accept the negative conclusions of review authors which, explicitly or implicitly, rested solely on such vote counts (without mentioning at least a moderate risk of bias) and b) that due to the almost exclusive RCT design the danger of false negativity was rated much higher than that of false positivity.[6]

This led to our three effectiveness categories:

1. Effectiveness likely, if in the domain analysis or the reviews studies could be found ($\geq$ 5% of the studies) with significant results in favour of homeopathy and with low risk of bias.[7]
2. Effectiveness questionable, if only non-significant results in favour of homeopathy were available or significant results with a moderate to high risk of bias.
3. Effectiveness unlikely, if no group difference could be detected in studies with a low risk of bias or if only studies with a high risk of bias showed a positive result.

For the clinical studies on the domain 'Upper Respiratory Tract Infection/ Allergy' (URTI/A), reanalysis with a view to external validity/relevance to practice generated the following result:

Evaluation of 29 systematically searched studies of different design (and EBM grading) on the domain 'Upper Respiratory Tract Infection/ Allergy' (URTI/A) showed an overall positive result in favour of homeopathy. 6 out of 7 of the controlled studies demonstrated at least equivalence with conventional medical interventions and 8 out of 16 placebo controlled studies significance in favour of homeopathy. This positive trend was maintained in the evaluation of subgroups.

Even considering the reduced external validity of randomized studies which is caused by their non practice-related methodology, the selection of study participants and blinding and which reduces their appropriateness in evaluating classical homeopathy, the study results still clearly demonstrate clinical efficacy for homeopathy. The positive effect is not only apparent in placebo controlled studies, but especially also in the comparison with conventional treatments.

---

6   It has to be added that academic convention fixed evaluation limits and recommendations for case number estimation in a way that minimizes the risk of false positive results – at $p \leq 0.05$ with a risk of c. 5% (although that cannot be fully maintained, cf. Niromaand 2004) – and the risk of false negative results at c. 20% – power of 80% – is considerably higher so that we gave more weight to significantly positive results in RCTs (which anyway tend towards false negative results) than to negative ones.

7   This descriptive method makes sense due to the heterogeneity of the studies and it basically corresponds to the procedure used by Kleijnen et al. (1991). It is still controversial seeing that systematic reviews and meta-analyses are carried out to avoid such estimations and to obtain more precise information concerning effectiveness. But it is exactly this precision of the meta-analysis that is questioned in the more recent discussion. Wegscheider (2005) explained that meta-analyses, unlike RCTs, are neither safe from overt nor from hidden bias, that the selection of their (statistical) units, the studies, is retrospective and very restrictive, that different endpoints and survey methods are used and that there is neither sample size planning nor confounder control. 'If one evaluated an RCT with these means, it would fail the Cochrane test'.

In the reviews, the demonstration of probable effectiveness is based on the four most extensive trials on the general effectiveness of homeopathy by Kleijnen (1991), Linde (1997 and 1998)
and Cucherat (2000). As our estimation of the risk of bias with regard to the real life healthcare
situation differs in some points from the conclusion of the authors, our rationale is again explained here:

1. Kleijnen et al. (1991) undertook the most comprehensive review of homeopathic literature
   so far with a three-year literature search. They found a total of 107 studies which they
   evaluated according to their own quality score with mostly internal validity criteria. Of the
   studies with the best quality (Score ≥ 55 of 100) 15 showed significant effects in favour of
   homeopathy, 7 did not. They concluded: The amount of positive evidence even among the
   best studies came as a surprise to us. Based on this evidence we would be ready to accept
   that homeopathy can be efficacious, if only the mechanism of action were more plausible.'
   As their reservations are only based on the plausibility issue, which we do not share in this
   form due to the preclinical research results known to us, we do not accept it and the result
   in favour of the effectiveness of homeopathy stands.

2. Linde 1997: 89 studies were submitted to a meta-analysis with an overall Odds Ratio (OR)
   of 2.45 (2.05–2.93 95% CI) in favour of homeopathy; for the 26 best studies an OR of 1.66
   (1.33–2.08 95% CI), after correction for publication bias: 1.78 (1.03–3.10 95% CI). The
   authors conclude: 'The results do not confirm the null hypothesis that there is no difference
   between homeopathy and placebo'. They do, however, qualify their evaluation because no
   definite evidence was found for the effectiveness of homeopathic medicines for a particular
   medical condition. The criticism of this study, which we share, was mainly that very heterogeneous data were summarized into an overall value. If one looks at the individual study
   results, almost half (18) of the 39 best quality studies (according to the Jadad Score or Linde's
   own score; with criteria of internal validity also predominating in the latter) find
   a significantly positive result in favour of homeopathy which means that a likely effectiveness for homeopathy can be concluded. The request for the consistency of study results for
   one particular condition arises out of the consideration that one needs studies that are comparable in at least one respect to determine whether a study result is accidentally or 'genuinely' positive. From the point of view of content it is not mandatory that the virtual entity
   of a conventional-medical disease picture should be the 'homogenizing' or 'moderating'
   (Walach) factor, although there might well be a subtle link between the symptoms and the
   organism's regulatory capacity.

3. Linde 1998: 19 clinical trials with individualized homeopathy were submitted to a meta-
   analysis and generated an overall OR of 1.62 (95% CI 1.17–2.23) but after restriction to the
   6 methodologically best studies the OR was non-significant at 1.12 (95% CI = 0.87–1.44).
   The authors concluded that homeopathic medicines probably have a greater effect than
   placebo, but that the evidence is not convincing due to the methodological quality of the
   studies. When the studies categorized as 'unlikely to have major flaws' (6 studies) were included in the consideration, the result was significant at 2.44 (95% CI 1.30–4.59).

4. Similar to the Cucherat (2000) trial which generated for 17 studies a combined p value of
   0.000036 (indicating the probability of at least one result not being accidentally positive)
   and only turned non significant after restriction to studies with a loss to follow-up ≤ 5% with
   p = 0.082, our evaluation of the Linde study can be controversially discussed:

In contrast to the now customary view that the reliability of results grows with internal validity,
we think that – roughly speaking – there is a risk of false positive results if the external validity

is overrated and a risk of false negative results if the internal validity is overrated. From the homeopathic point of view, the external validity is low with most studies (apart from the newer, more practice related outcome studies) because they tend to ignore the essential foundations of classical homeopathy. When we looked for a threshold from which the internal validity of studies was considered to be 'good', we found a few variations (e.g. Kleijnen: ≥ 55 out of 100 based on their own score; Ernst: ≥ 90 out of 100; classification in low, moderate, high risk of bias; setting the bias threshold for drop-outs not, as is usually done, at 10%, but at 5% as Cucherat does or 20% as in SIGN 50). In order not to create an arbitrary threshold, but also not to blindly adhere to the 'the more internally valid, the better' tenet we decided, based on the Cochrane Handbook 2001, in favour of the three-stage classification into low, moderate and high risk of bias and also retained the bias threshold of 10% lost to follow-up. This resulted in our assumption that a) the category 'unlikely to have major flaws' in the Linde study was included in the evaluation as probably carrying a low risk of bias and that b) the significant result of the Cucherat study with 10% lost to follow-up had been used as a basis and that therefore both review results were classified as 'likely to be effective' for homeopathy.

From the homeopathic point of view the positive result of the investigations available is remarkable because a number of comprehensive surveys, the majority of which yielded definitely positive results in favour of homeopathy, do not even figure in this analysis because they do not meet the criteria of a systematic review. A study – conducted and published as part of the PEK programme – on the quality and results of homeopathic trials in comparison to conventional medical trials, which gave rise to heated discussion (Shang et al. 2005), has been largely invalidated by the research of Lüdtke & Rutten (2008) and Rutten & Stolper (2008).

As mentioned above, the evaluation of effectiveness was considered in great detail as it continues to be put into question because its mode of action cannot be explained. It certainly is an important basis for the estimation of cost effectiveness, demand and supply, as the use of inexpensive therapies does not make sense if they produce no effect.

Concerning the evaluation of safety, use and cost effectiveness of homeopathy the following results were established:

Medical homeopathy is of a high standard in Switzerland and was up to the year 2005 covered by the Swiss statutory health insurance alongside conventional medical methods. Provision of homeopathic healthcare is not adequate, especially not in rural areas. Even in towns where provision is good demand exceeds supply which can manifest in long waiting lists.

The supply of medicines is regulated by *swissmedic* (formerly IKS) and basically covered by manufacturers in Switzerland. Recently introduced regulations on expiry dates and biological safety are a threat to the homeopathic stock of medicines.

Homeopathy does not have enough academic presence (only a quarter professorship at Berne University), especially as the chair is underequipped for teaching and research and there is no large scale industrial support.

■ Safety

The Swiss regulations guarantee a high degree of safety as training requirements for homeopathic physicians and product regulations are very strict. There is, if anything, a danger of over-regimentation. The frequently described 'main complication' of homeopathy, i.e. the omission of other meaningful treatments, is not to be expected because of the high-standard qualification for physicians (corresponding to the strict training requirements). Medical homeopathy in Switzerland has few side effects if professionally executed and the use of high potencies is free from toxic effects.

■ **Appropriateness**

Appropriateness is divided into two sections: demand/use and safety. For both the relevant literature was found mainly through expert contacts and the search of bibliographical references.

The material yielded the following information: About half of the Swiss population has used CAM and values it. About half the physicians, the great majority of CAM users and c. 40% of cancer patients consider CAM to be effective. The major part of the population (≥ 50%) would prefer a CAM hospital. A great majority (85%) of the population would wish for CAM to be included in the national health insurance scheme (Jenny et al. 2002). International studies also show that the use of CAM therapies in the countries investigated (mostly USA, UK, Germany, France) is not just a marginal phenomenon, but has been steadily increasing over the years.

■ **Economy**

There are few data from health economic studies on individual specialties. They are mostly investigated under the umbrella of 'complementary alternative medicine' (CAM), an area that is mostly very broadly defined (e.g. diet and physical measures). There are several studies on homeopathy from Germany, England and France which confirm good cost effectiveness of the methods used. The largest survey which was carried out by a French social insurance provider underlines the low costs of homeopathy (Chaufferin 2000, Taieb & Myon 2003, Trichard et al. 2003). There are more comprehensive studies on several CAM specialties from Germany (pilot projects of health insurance companies, Marstedt & Moebus 2002) and one study from Switzerland (Sommer et al. 1999). The Swiss study inferred an additive and possibly cost increasing effect of including CAM into statutory healthcare provision, giving rise to widespread discussion (Heusser 1999, Kienle & Kiene 1999). Points of criticism refer mostly to structural aspects and seriously question the conclusions drawn by the authors from the collected data. Doubts relate in particular to the comparability of the groups with regard to the insurance holders' state of health at study begin and the possible use of CAM in the comparison group from year 2 of the trial. Further restrictions apply due to the small number of patients evaluated (some groups with less than 10 patients) and the assessment of the quality of life over the phone.

The now published results of the German pilot projects (Güthlin & Walach 2001, Güthlin et al. 2004) which used a provision research approach similar to that of the Swiss study, indicate sustained effectiveness of CAM therapies with possible cost savings: two pilot projects showed a definite and sustained decrease in sick leave days before and after treatment begin from 32 before to 23 or 24 days in the second observation year. Data concerning direct costs cannot be extracted from the pilot projects.

The economic aspects of homeopathy have been increasingly scrutinized in recent years. Apart from studies and other surveys, more and more comments and summaries on the subject are published in various journals: Schüppel et al. (2003) conclude from a review of the published data that, with pharmaceutical costs being what they are, the use of homeopathy has the potential to lower pharmaceutical spending. Whether the costs per case remain lower than for conventional medicine on the long term has to be established by further studies with longer observation periods.

A general health economic conclusion for homeopathy as a system cannot be drawn from the data available. Individual studies, such as the German health insurance pilot projects, confirm sustained effectiveness and thus potential savings of indirect costs, measured in a reduction of days off work due to sickness.

In summary it can be said that there is sufficient evidence for the preclinical (experimental) effectiveness and the clinical efficacy of homeopathy and for its safety and economy compared to conventional treatment. It is a highly popular intervention. From the homeopathic point of view, the positive evidence with regard to its action and effectiveness is the more remarkable as most research studies violate its fundamental rules. In the interest of scientific recognition, external evidence is often sacrificed for the sake of internal validity which leads to the risk of false negative results. Future research methods must respect the unique qualities of homeopathy by attaching more weight to single case evaluations, by including practically and expertly applied homeopathic treatment into research and clinical practice in order to identify its real potential and limitations. The recently introduced outcome studies are promising in this respect as they do not focus on specific effect but on the overall practical treatment and patient care in homeopathy.

13.1   References

Alderson P, Green S, Higgins J. Cochrane Reviewers' Handbook. Handbook 4.2.1. [updated December 2003]. Chichester: John Wiley & Sons Ltd, 2004

Altman DG, Bland JM. Absence of evidence is not evidence of absence. British Medical Journal 1995;311:485

Chaufferin G. Improving the evaluation of homeopathy: economic considerations and impact on health. British Homeopathic Journal 2000;89(1):27–30

Cucherat M, Haugh MC, Gooch M, Boissel JP. Evidence of clinical efficacy of homeopathy (A meta-analysis of clinical trials). European Journal of Clinical Pharmacology 2000;56:27–33

Glanville J, Sowden A. Identification of the need for a review. In: Khan K, ter Riet G, Glanville J, Sowden A, Kleijnen J (editors). Undertaking Systematic Reviews of Research on Effectiveness. CRD Report Number 4 (2nd Edition), York, 2001

Güthlin C, Walach H. Prospektive Dokumentationsstudie in der niedergelassenen Praxis – ein Erprobungsverfahren zur Akupunktur und Homöopathie. Erfahrungsheilkunde 2001;(50):186–94

Güthlin C, Lange O, Walach H. Measuring the effects of acupuncture and homeopathy in general practice: An uncontrolled prospective documentation approach. BMC Public Health 2004;4(6).

Heusser P. Komplementärmedizin in der Grundversicherung: Verteuert sie die Gesundheitskosten? Schweizerische Zeitschrift für GanzheitsMedizin 1999;11:4–9

Jenny S, Simon M, Meier B. Haltung der Bevölkerung gegenüber der Komplementärmedizin Schweizerische Zeitschrift für GanzheitsMedizin 2002;14:340–7

Kienle G. Arzneimittelsicherheit und Gesellschaft. Eine kritische Untersuchung. Stuttgart New York: Schattauer, 1974

Kienle GS, Kiene H. Können aus der Studie „Komplementärmedizin in der Krankenversicherung" wissenschaftlich tragfähige Schlüsse gezogen werden? Forschende Komplementärmedizin 1999;6(5):262–70

Kienle GS, Kiene H, Albonico HU. Anthroposophic Medicine. Effectiveness, utility, costs, safety. Stuttgart New York: Schattauer 2006b

Kleijnen J, Knipschild P, ter Riet G. Clinical trials of homeopathy. British Medical Journal 1991;302(6772):316–23.

Linde K, Clausius N, Ramirez G, Melchart D, Eitel F, Hedges LV, Jonas WB. Are the clinical effects of homeopathy placebo effects? A meta-analysis of placebo-controlled trials. Lancet 1997;350(9081):834–43.

Linde K, Melchart D: Randomized controlled trials of individual homeopathy: a state-of-the-art review. The Journal of Alternative and Complementary Medicine 1998;4(4):371–388

Lüdtke R, Rutten ALB. The conclusions on the effectiveness of homeopathy highly depend on the set of analyzed trials. Journal of Clinical Epidemiology. 2008; 61(12):1197–1204.

Marstedt G, Moebus S. Gesundheitsberichterstattung des Bundes Heft 9: Inanspruchnahme alternativer Methoden in der Medizin. Berlin: Verlag Robert Koch Institut, 2002

Mathie RT: The research ecidence base for homeopathy: a fresh assessment of the literature. Homeopathy 2003; 92(2):84–91

Niroomand F. Evidenzbasierte Medizin: Das Individuum bleibt auf der Strecke. Deutsches Ärzteblatt 2004; 101(26):1870–4

Rutten AL, Stolper, CF. The 2005 meta-analysis of homeopathy: the importance of post-publication data. Homeopathy. 2008;97(4):169–77

Schüppel R. Kosten und Nutzen der Homöopathie - Ein echtes Schnäppchen? Der Hausarzt 2003;19:64

Shang A, Huwiler-Muntener K, Nartey L et al. Are the clinical effects of homoeopathy placebo effects? Comparative study of placebo-controlled trials of homoeopathy and allopathy. Lancet 2005; 366: 726–732

SIGN 50 (Scottish Intercollegiate Guidelines Network). A guideline developer's handbook. Notes on the use of Methodology Checklist 2: Randomized Controlled Trials. 2005. available at: http://www.sign.ac.uk/guidelines/fulltext/50/notes2.html

Sommer JH, Burgi M, Theiss R. Inclusion of complementary medicine increases health costs. Focus on Alternative & Complementary Therapies 1999;4(4):183–4

Taieb C, Myon E. The economic impact of homeopathic management: the french example. Value Health 2003; 6(3):373

Trichard M, Chaufferin G, Nicoloyannis N. Pharmacoeconomic comparison between two drug stragegies of treatment of anxiety disorders: homeopathy and psychotropics (ISPOR Poster PMH23). Value in Health 2003; 6(3):350–1

Walach H. Unspezifische Therapie-Effekte – Das Beispiel Homöopathie. Habilitationsschrift Psychologisches Institut, Albert-Ludwigs-Universität Freiburg, 1997

Wegscheider K. Was sind faire Vergleiche zwischen Therapien? Zeitschrift für ärztliche Fortbildung und Qualität im Gesundheitswesen 2005;99(4–5):275–8

Wein C. Qualitätsaspekte klinischer Studien zur Homöopathie. Essen: KVC-Verlag, 2002

World Medical Association, Declaration of Helsinki. Ethical principles for medical research involving human subjects. Bulletin of the World Health Organization, 2001;79(4):373-4. available at: http://whqlibdoc.who.int/bulletin/2001/issue4/79(4)declaration.pdf

13

Synopsis

This Health Technology Assessment (HTA) report was compiled on behalf of the Swiss Federal Social Insurance Office as part of the Complementary Medicine Evaluation Project (PEK) in order to evaluate the speciality homeopathy (alongside four other complementary medical methods: phytotherapy, neural therapy, anthroposophically extended medicine and traditional Chinese medicine – phytotherapy) for their efficacy, appropriateness and cost-effectiveness. Next to the primary study carried out by the PEK, the HTA report was to provide the basis for the decision whether statutory health insurance compensation should continue beyond 30 June 2006.

The literature for this HTA report was retrieved from internet-accessible databases such as Medline, Embase, Amed, Mantis, PsycInfo, Econlit and others and, as this did not prove sufficient, also via expert contacts and the search through bibliographical references. Data extraction was carried out via specially designed questionnaires which conform to international recommendations regarding the compilation of HTAs while also reflecting criteria of external validity.

The individual research questions and results were as follows:

14.1 Effectiveness

For the evaluation of the effectiveness of homeopathy all available systematic reviews were examined and the literature on a particular indication (upper respiratory tract infections/allergy – URTI) was analysed for all study designs.

14.2 Reviews

All systematic reviews relating to homeopathy (as a system or to individual indications and interventions) which were completed and available by June 2003 were analysed for their internal as well as external validity. The following inclusion criteria applied: study design, i.e. systematic review or meta-analysis with the criteria: systematic search in adequate databases (at least Medline) with information on inclusion and exclusion criteria or the explicit statement that a systematic search had been conducted. Publication was a further prerequisite. Exclusion criteria: failure to meet the inclusion criteria, e.g. no systematic review or review on drug tests, research questions that were irrelevant to our HTA, reanalyses, i.e. articles that re-evaluate other reviews (these reanalyses were included as comments with the presentation of the corresponding original reviews), double publications.

A total of 22 reviews were analysed. The majority (ten of 22, with 563 analysed studies in total) examined homeopathy as a therapy system, seven the effectiveness of homeopathy for particular medical conditions, three a specific homeopathic medicine (Arnica), and two a particular homeopathic remedy with a particular medical condition.

The synopsis of study results found at least a trend in favour of homeopathy in 20 of 22 reviews. The results of five of these literature studies clearly supported the effectiveness of a homeopathic intervention in our estimation; four of them investigated the effectiveness of homeopathy as a therapy system, among them the very controversial study by Linde et al. (1997). A follow-up study with very high external validity, i.e. the investigation of the effectiveness of individualized classical homeopathy, also provided strong evidence of effectiveness. The fifth study focused on a defined acute clinical condition, post-operative ileus, where homeopathic medicines produced results that were statistically significant as well as clinically relevant.

In two (of 22) reviews no positive proof of effectiveness was established for the homeopathic treatment.

Final conclusion after analysis of the reviews on homeopathy: in a three-tier evaluation scale of the 'real-world effectiveness' (effectiveness likely, questionable or unlikely)', homeopathy falls within the category: 'effectiveness likely'.

14.3 Studies on the Indication Upper Respiratory Tract Infection/ Allergy (URTI/A)

As almost all reviews included only randomized studies – which carry a risk of bias with regard to external validity and are therefore not adequate for the evaluation of health-care provision in everyday practice – we investigated all studies that focused on a particular indication ('domain': infections of the upper respiratory tract). Twenty-nine trials were analysed; 17 of them were RCTs (EBM evidence grade 1b), six were controlled trials without randomisation (EBM evidence grade 2a), four were observational studies with control (EBM evidence grade 2b), one was a retrospective cohort study (EBM evidence grade 3) and one a single case report (EBM evidence grade 4). Evaluation of the studies produced an overall positive result for 24 of the 29 studies investigated. This positive trend was upheld in the evaluation of certain subgroups. If one considers only the placebo-controlled, randomized studies with the highest EBM grading, 12 of 16 studies show a positive result for the homeopathically treated group (significantly positive 8/16 and trend 4/16). The comparison to conventional treatment shows a positive result in 6/7 studies (significantly positive 1/7 and equivalence with conventional treatment 5/7).

The overall conclusion was: internal as well as external validity and therefore also the transferability of results to the situation in Switzerland are restricted due to various aspects which, however, do not put in question the fundamental effectiveness of homeopathic treatment in clinical reality. Independent of the study design, the study results showed a probable effectiveness of homeopathy for allergies and upper respiratory tract infections. Tolerability is very good and also not restricted when combined with conventional treatment. There could be economic advantages due to the fact that the homeopathic treatment can reduce the need for conventional medication.

The homeopathic side points out that only very few of the studies analysed for the HTA are relevant to homeopathic practice and to the internal homeopathic research that is practice related. From the homeopathic point of view such studies are therefore ambiguous: they can, as is shown here, testify the effectiveness of homeopathic methods, but they (especially, and paradoxically, those that provide the strongest evidence) present homeopathy 'distorted' through being forced into study designs that are alien to homeopathic practice and methodology and do not reflect the real situation (low external and model validity). They are 'justification research', conducted with a view to gaining scientific and political recognition for homeopathy, but they are hardly significant and therefore of little interest to homeopaths. The newer provision studies of recent years have developed methods that are less biased and more practice related (individualized homeopathy, longer observation periods) and therefore more suitable to evaluate homeopathic medicine.

14.4   Appropriateness

Appropriateness is divided into two areas – demand/use and safety. For both, the relevant literature was retrieved mostly via expert contacts and the study of bibliographical references.

14.4.1 Estimation of Demand/Use

Most studies examined the general utilisation of CAM therapies (CAM: complementary and alternative medicine) without singling out individual methods such as homeopathy. A total of 52 studies of utilisation were found in the international literature; for Switzerland in particular 20 studies were evaluated. The material revealed that about half of the Swiss population uses CAM and appreciates it (this corresponds largely to the international data). About half the physicians, the great majority of CAM users and ca. 40% of cancer patients consider it to be effective. A large part of the population (≥50%) would prefer a CAM hospital to one with conventional orientation. A vast majority (85%) of the population wish for CAM to be included in the statutory health-care provision. International studies also show that the use of CAM therapies is more than a marginal phenomenon in the countries investigated (mostly USA, UK, Germany, France etc.) and that its use has been increasing over the years.

14.4.2 Safety

The Swiss regulations guarantee a high degree of safety as training requirements for homeopathic physicians, and product regulations are very strict. There is, if anything, a danger of over-regimentation. The frequently described 'main complication' of homeopathy, i.e. the omission of other meaningful treatments, is not to be expected because of the high-standard qualification for physicians. Medical homeopathy in Switzerland has few side effects if professionally executed, and the use of high potencies is free from toxic effects.

14.5   Economy

There are few data from health economic studies on individual specialities. They are investigated mostly under the umbrella of 'complementary alternative medicine' (CAM), an area that is usually very broadly defined (e.g. diet and physical measures). For homeopathy the study situation is still very favourable. There are several studies on homeopathy from Germany, England and France which confirm good cost-effectiveness of the methods used. The largest survey which was carried out by a French social insurance provider underlines the low costs of homeopathy.

There are more comprehensive studies on several CAM specialities from Germany (pilot projects of health insurance companies) and one study from Switzerland (Sommer et al. 1999). The Swiss study inferred an additive and possibly cost-increasing effect of including CAM into statutory health-care provision, giving rise to widespread discussion. Points of criticism refer mostly to structural aspects and seriously question the conclusions drawn by the authors from the collected data.

Doubts relate in particular to the comparability of the groups with regard to the insurance holders' state of health at study begin and the possible use of CAM in the comparison group from year 2 of the trial. Further restrictions apply due to the small number of patients evaluated (some groups with fewer than ten patients) and the assessment of the quality of life over the phone.

The now published results of the German pilot projects, which used a provision research approach similar to that of the Swiss study, indicate sustained effectiveness of CAM therapies with possible cost savings: two pilot projects showed a definite and sustained decrease in sick-leave days before and after treatment begin from 32 before to 23 or 24 days in the second observation year. Data concerning direct costs cannot be extracted from the pilot projects.

The economic aspects of homeopathy have been increasingly scrutinized in recent years. Apart from studies and other surveys, more and more comments and summaries on the subject are being published in various journals: Schüppel et al. (2003) conclude from a review of the published data that, with pharmaceutical costs being what they are, the use of homeopathy has the potential to lower pharmaceutical spending. Whether the costs per case remain lower than for conventional medicine in the long term has to be established by further studies with longer observation periods.

A general health-economic conclusion for homeopathy as a system cannot be drawn from the data available. Individual studies, such as the German health insurance pilot projects, confirm sustained effectiveness and thus potential savings in indirect costs, measured in the reduction of days off work due to sickness.

In summary, it can be said that there is sufficient evidence for the preclinical effectiveness and the clinical efficacy of homeopathy (evidence grades I and II) and for its safety and economy compared with conventional treatment. It is a highly popular intervention. Future research methods must respect the unique qualities of homeopathy by attaching more weight to single case evaluations, by including practically and expertly applied homeopathic treatment into research and clinical practice in order to identify its real potential and limitations.

In spite of these positive results the Swiss Federal Office of Public Health[1] decided to withdraw homeopathy from the list of services covered by the national statutory health insurance.

However, in a referendum of 17 May 2009, the great majority of the Swiss population voted for complementary medicine to be integrated in the national health system. The following amendment was added to the constitution: 'The Federal Government and Cantons shall ensure that, within the scope of their jurisdiction, complementary medicine is taken into consideration.'

In January 2011 the Swiss Federal Department of Home Affairs[2] decided that as of 1 January 2012 homeopathy will, among others, be included in the Swiss statutory health insurance and reimbursed for a minimum of 6 years.

---

1   Schweizer Bundesamt für Gesundheit (BAG)
2   Eidgenössisches Department des Inneren (EDI)

Appendix

15

15.1 Data Extraction Forms – 212

15.1.1 Sample questionnaires: systematic reviews and meta-analyses, also for HTA – 212

15.1.2 Sample questionnaires: clinical studies – 218

15.1.3 Sample questionnaire: demand/cost-effectiveness – 224

15.2 Abbreviations – 227

15.3 Conflict of interest – 230

15.4 Authors – 230

15.1   Data Extraction Forms

15.1.1 Sample questionnaires: systematic reviews and meta-analyses, also for HTA

The following tables are questionnaires for data extraction and for the evaluation of full-text articles or other publications, design: HTA, meta-analysis or systematic review. Some questions apply only to HTAs.

■ Table 15.1 General information (publication and reviewer)

Question	Answer
Author	
Year of publication	
Title	
Data source	☐ database, Internet (systematic search) ☐ database, not publically accessible ☐ hand search (systematic search) ☐ personal contacts (no systematic search) ☐ not known to reviewer
Speciality	☐ homeopathy ☐ phytotherapy ☐ TCM ☐ neural therapy ☐ anthroposophy
Type of publication	☐ abstract ☐ congress presentation ☐ full text article ☐ letter ☐ short report ☐ thesis ☐ book ☐ presentation ☐ other/(not published)
Language	☐ English ☐ German ☐ Chinese ☐ Italian ☐ French ☐ other:
Reviewer	
Date	

15

Table 15.2 Background: research question and context of HTA/systematic reviews

Question	Answer		
Is the context for commissioning the HTA documented?	☐ yes	☐ no	☐ not applicable
Is a reason documented for carrying out the HTA?	☐ yes	☐ no	
Is the decision documented which the HTA is meant to support?	☐ yes	☐ no	
Is the time frame of the HTA documented?	☐ yes	☐ no	
Please state time frame of HTA:			
Is a clear research question documented?	☐ yes	☐ no	
Please state HTA question(s): (key words):			
If applicable: Please state medical condition/indication investigated in the article:	☐ not applicable		
If applicable: Please state intervention/medication/type of therapy investigated in the article:	☐ not applicable		
Is the question relevant to the decision which the HTA is meant to support?	☐ relevant ☐ not relevant	☐ partly relevant ☐ ?	
Is the HTA question relevant to the decision which the HTA is meant to support?	☐ relevant ☐ not relevant	☐ partly relevant ☐ ?	
Comment on external validity of HTA/review question			

Table 15.3 Methodological aspects and information capture

Question	Answer	
Was an HTA protocol prepared?	☐ yes ☐ no ☐ not documented	
Are reasons documented if HTA protocol was not adhered to?	☐ yes	☐ no
Reasons for non-adherence to protocol:		
Is the method of identifying data sources documented?	☐ yes	☐ no
Is there documentation of the sources used?	☐ yes ☐ partly	☐ yes, but not in the article ☐ no
Please name the databases used:		
Are the search strategies documented? ▼	☐ yes ☐ partly	☐ yes, but not in the article ☐ no

▣ Table 15.3 (continued)

Question	Answer	
Is the time of the database access documented?	☐ yes ☐ no	☐ partly
Was preselection carried out by several reviewers independently?	☐ yes ☐ no	☐ partly ☐ not documented
Are the criteria for the qualitative evaluation of studies documented?	☐ yes ☐ no	☐ partly
Are inclusion criteria for the studies documented?	☐ yes ☐ no	☐ partly
Please state inclusion criteria:		
Are the exclusion criteria for the studies documented?	☐ yes ☐ no	☐ partly
Please state exclusion criteria		
Are excluded studies documented, with reasons for exclusion?	☐ yes ☐ partly	☐ yes, but not in the article ☐ no
Are possible bias factors of included primary studies documented?	☐ yes	☐ partly ☐ no
Was data extraction/evaluation carried out by several reviewers independently?	☐ yes ☐ no	☐ partly ☐ not documented
Did an external review take place?	☐ yes	☐ no
Funding	☐ sponsor named	☐ not named
Overall evaluation: Are identification/selection and extraction of data clearly and adequately documented?	☐ adequate ☐ not adequate	☐ partly adequate ☐ ?
Comment on overall evaluation of data identification/selection and extraction:		
Is the research question adequate (correct, suitable) to support the HTA decision?	☐ adequate ☐ not adequate	☐ partly adequate ☐ ?
Is the research question relevant to the question of this particular study?	☐ relevant ☐ not relevant	☐ partly relevant ☐ ?
Comment on relevance of research question to this study		

15

■ **Table 15.4** Information synthesis

Question	Answer
Was a quantitative information synthesis carried out?	☐ yes ☐ no ☐ not documented
Is the meta-analysis method documented?	☐ documented ☐ partly documented ☐ not documented
Were heterogeneity tests carried out?	☐ yes ☐ no ☐ not documented
Were other quantitative procedures carried out?	☐ yes ☐ no ☐ not documented
If yes: please state which quantitative procedures were carried out:	
Were the results tested for robustness in a sensitivity analysis?	☐ yes ☐ no ☐ not documented
Was a qualitative information synthesis carried out?	☐ yes ☐ no ☐ not documented
Please give more details of qualitative information analysis.	
Is the information synthesis method adequately documented?	☐ adequate ☐ adequate to an extent ☐ not adequate
Are the data synthesis methods adequate for answering the review/HTA question?	☐ adequate ☐ partly adequate ☐ not adequate ☐ ?
Comments on data synthesis method (internal validity):	
Are the data synthesis methods relevant for answering the research question of this particular study?	☐ relevant ☐ relevant to an extent ☐ not relevant ☐ ?
Comments on data synthesis method (external validity):	

◘ Table 15.5 Methods and results

Question	Answer
Is the answer to the review/HTA question documented?	☐ yes ☐ partly ☐ no
Please give a brief summary of the answer to the research question.	
Are methodical limitations to the relevance critically documented?	☐ documented ☐ not documented
Are there recommendations for further action?	☐ yes ☐ no ☐ not documented
Are the recommendations graded?	☐ yes ☐ no ☐ not documented
Was the need for further research identified?	☐ yes ☐ no ☐ not documented
Is a review update envisaged?	☐ yes ☐ no ☐ not documented
Is the evidence established adequately (=logically) reflected in the final conclusions?	☐ adequate ☐ adequate to an extent ☐ not adequate ☐ ?
Is the way in which the evidence established is reflected in the HTA's final conclusions relevant to research question of this particular study?	☐ relevant ☐ relevant to an extent ☐ not relevant ☐ ?
Comments on how evidence is reflected in final conclusions:	

◘ Table 15.6 HTA/review technique. Transferability of international/foreign results and final conclusions (external validity)

Question	Answer
Is the technique documented for the country that is relevant to the HTA?	☐ yes ☐ no
Comments:	
Are aspects documented that could influence the transfer of results from other countries to the country under consideration?	☐ yes ☐ no
Is the description of results adequate for the country relevant to the HTA?	☐ adequate ☐ partly adequate ☐ not adequate ☐ ?
Is the technique documented in a way that is useful/transferable to the country relevant to question of this particular study? ▼	☐ relevant ☐ relevant to an extent ☐ not relevant ☐ ?

15

▣ Table 15.6 (continued)

Question	Answer	
Is the discussion of transferability aspects adequate with regard to the HTA question?	☐ adequate ☐ not adequate	☐ adequate to an extent ☐ ?
Is the discussion of transferability aspects relevant with regard to the question of this study?	☐ relevant ☐ not relevant	☐ partly relevant ☐ ?

▣ Table 15.7 Evaluation/recommendation

Question	Answer		
Author: advantage (discussion part)	☐ yes ☐ partly ☐ no ☐ not documented		
Author: comment			
Are potential bias factors adequately considered?	☐ adequate ☐ not adequate	☐ partly adequate ☐ ?	
Comments on evaluation of bias factors			
Reviewer: advantage	☐ yes	☐ to an extent	☐ no
Reviewer: estimation of effectiveness	☐ effectiveness likely ☐ effectiveness questionable ☐ effectiveness unlikely ☐ not documented		
Comment on estimated effectiveness			
Reviewer: estimated appropriateness (risks, safety etc.)	risk: ☐ slight ☐ medium ☐ severe (hospitalisation, lasting hereditary damage, death, danger of death) ☐ not documented		
Comment on estimation of appropriateness:			
Reviewer: estimation of cost-effectiveness (compared with control intervention):	☐ higher effectiveness, higher costs lower effectiveness, higher costs ☐ lower effectiveness, lower costs ☐ higher effectiveness, lower costs ☐ not documented		
Comment on estimation of cost-effectiveness			
Reviewer: general rationale/comments on article			
Is the article relevant for the speciality in Switzerland?	☐ relevant ☐ not relevant	☐ relevant to an extent	

15.1.2 **Sample questionnaires: clinical studies**

▣ Table 15.8 General information

Question	Answer
Author	
Year of publication	
Title	
Data sources	☐ database, internet (systematic search) ☐ database, not publically accessible ☐ hand search (systematic search) ☐ personal contacts (no systematic search) ☐ not known to reviewer
Article on Medline index?	☐ yes ☐ no ☐ ?
Type of publication	☐ abstract ☐ congress presentation ☐ full text article ☐ letter ☐ short report ☐ thesis ☐ book ☐ presentation ☐ other (not published)
Language	
Country	
Reviewer	
Date	
Design (category)	☐ RCT ☐ CT ☐ matched pair analysis ☐ cohort study (longitudinal) ☐ cross-sectional ☐ other, please state:

▣ Table 15.9 Research question of trial

Question	Answer
Research question	
Research question adequate (clear, reproducible)?	☐ yes ☐ partly ☐ no comment:
Research question relevant to the question of this particular study (external validity)?	☐ yes ☐ partly ☐ no ☐ ? comment:

15

□ Table 15.10 Population

Question	Answer
Main diagnosis/indication:	.... comment (duration and severity as well as co-morbidities and prognostic factors stated?):
Was the diagnosis correctly established in conventional medical terms?	☐ yes ☐ partly ☐ no ☐ n.a.
How was the (conventional medical) diagnosis established?	☐ history-taking ☐ clinical examination ☐ laboratory ☐ instrument-based ☐ other
Was the diagnosis established in a way that is compatible with the speciality?	☐ yes ☐ no ☐ n/a
Basic overall study population[1]	.... comment (relevance of population for indication):
Inclusion criteria:	
Exclusion criteria:	
Number of participants at trial begin (n)[2]	
Male/female ratio	
Age of participants at trial begin?	mean value ± SD
Most important characteristics adequately documented at trial begin?	☐ yes ☐ partly ☐ no ☐ n.a. ☐ not documented
Groups comparable at trial begin (selection bias)?	☐ yes ☐ partly ☐ no comment:
Adjuvant medication (during trial)?	comment:
Is the population relevant with regard to the question of this particular study?	☐ yes ☐ partly ☐ no ☐ not clear comment:

1 Description of patient group from which study participants were recruited, e.g. oncology outpatients, university hospital; primary school etc.
2 Number of randomized patients (not number of patients questioned/screened!)

Table 15.11 Study design/methods

Question	Answer
Detailed description of study design:	☐ double blinding (physician + patient) ☐ simple blinding (patient only) ☐ randomized ☐ controlled ☐ case control study ☐ with matching ☐ without matching ☐ one group/cohort ☐ several groups/cohorts ☐ retrospective ☐ prospective ☐ n/a
Randomisation method adequate? ('random sequence generation')	☐ yes ☐ partly ☐ no ☐ n.a. ☐ not documented
Blinding method adequate (physician, patient)?	☐ yes ☐ partly ☐ no ☐ n.a. ☐ not documented
Design adequate (internal validity, performance bias)?	☐ yes ☐ partly ☐ no ☐ not clear comment:
Study design adequate for speciality (external validity)	☐ yes ☐ partly ☐ no ☐ not clear ☐ comment:

Table 15.12 Intervention

Question	Answer
Main intervention (state name of medication)	
How many groups are there in the study?	
Control intervention/s	☐ placebo others:
Total length of treatment	
Intervention adequately (clearly) documented (internal validity), reproducibility?	☐ yes ☐ partly ☐ no ☐ ? comment (performance bias):
Intervention carried out correctly (in line with speciality)?	☐ yes ☐ partly ☐ no ☐ ? comment:

15

▣ Table 15.13 Outcome and results

Question	Answer
Were one or more main end points predefined?	☐ yes ☐ no ☐ not documented
State main end point/s:	
How many secondary end points were assessed/defined?	
State secondary end points:	
Classification of main end point	☐ surrogate parameter ☐ clinical parameter ☐ quality of life ☐ clinical parameter + surrogate parameter ☐ clinical parameter + quality of life ☐ other combinations cost effectiveness
How was the end point determined?	+ comments:
Are the values for the main outcome parameter adequately documented?	☐ yes ☐ partly ☐ no ☐ ? comment:
End point relevant for medical condition under investigation?	☐ yes ☐ to an extent ☐ no ☐ ?
Number of treated persons per group	
Number of evaluated patients per group (if different from number of persons treated)	
Documentation of adverse effects/unexpected adverse events (UAE) adequate?	☐ yes ☐ to an extent ☐ no ☐ not documented
Documentation of withdrawals and lost to follow-up adequate?	☐ yes ☐ to an extent ☐ no ☐ not documented comment (attrition bias):
Comment on end point determination (measuring method: validity and significance of end point)	

Four field table (main target parameters)

	verum	control
successful		
not successful		

Results for primary parameters

++ statistical significance (for the treatment)
+ trend for the treatment
+/- no difference
- trend for control treatment
-- statistical significance for control treatment

▼

◘ Table 15.13 (continued)

Question	Answer
Results for secondary parameters	++ statistical significance (for the treatment) + trend for treatment +/- no difference - trend for control treatment -- statistical significance for control treatment not documented
Results for side effects and unexpected adverse events (UAE)	++ statistical significance (for the treatment) + trend for treatment +/- no difference - trend for control treatment -- statistical significance for control treatment Ø no side effects observed not documented

◘ Table 15.14 Statistics (analyses)

Question	Answer	
Which statistical tests were used to analyse results? Please state names:		
Type of analysis	☐ ITT ☐ not doc.	☐ PP ☐ other; please state:
Was it taken into account for the analysis if groups were not comparable at baseline? (adjustment)	☐ yes ☐ not documented	☐ no ☐ n.a.
Which group was advantaged by non-adjustment?	☐ verum group ☐ n.a.	☐ control group ☐ ?
How is the statistical analysis of main outcome parameters documented?	☐ test statistics and p-values documented ☐ p-level doc., test statistics values not doc. ☐ test statistics doc., p-value not documented ☐ no test statistics nor p-value stated ☐ other information (comment to be entered under detection bias!)	
Overall evaluation: statistical analysis adequate?	☐ yes ☐ no	☐ partly ☐ not evaluable
Detection bias:	comments:	
ITT = intention to treat (-analysis), PP = per protocol (-analysis)		

15

■ Table 15.15 Questions specific to homeopathy

Question	Answer
Treatment according to similarity rule	☐ yes ☐ to an extent (e.g. complex remedy) ☐ no ☐ not documented
Treatment concept	☐ individual homeopathy ☐ clinical homeopathy ☐ complex homeopathy ☐ isopathy ☐ not documented
Validation of symptoms (hierarchisation/repertorisation) documented	☐ yes ☐ no
Confounding factors considered?	☐ yes ☐ no
Were homeopathic reactions and results evaluated in line with homeopathic criteria?	☐ yes ☐ no
Comments: (aspects of specialist method)	

■ Table 15.16 Evaluation/recommendation

Question	Answer
Author: advantage (discussion)	☐ yes ☐ to an extent ☐ no ☐ not documented author's comments:
Reviewer: estimated effectiveness	☐ effectiveness likely ☐ effectiveness questionable ☐ effectiveness unlikely
Reviewer: estimation of appropriateness (risks, safety etc.)	risk: ☐ practically no risks ☐ slight ☐ medium ☐ severe (hospitalisation, lasting hereditary damage, death , danger of death) ☐ not documented
Reviewer: general comments	

■ Table 15.17 Overall evaluation

	good (+)	medium (+/–)	poor (–)
Article: [author, publication year + short title]			
Documentation (level 1)			
Internal validity (level 2)			
External validity (level 3)			

15.1.3 **Sample questionnaire: demand/cost-effectiveness**

▫ Table 15.18 General information (publication and reviewer)

Question	Answer	
Author		
Year of publication		
Title		
Source of data	☐ database, internet (systematic search) ☐ database, not publically accessible ☐ hand search (systematic search) ☐ personal contacts (no systematic search) ☐ not known to reviewer	
Type of publication	☐ abstract ☐ full text article ☐ short report ☐ book ☐ other/(not published)	☐ congress presentation ☐ letter ☐ thesis ☐ presentation
Country	☐ Germany ☐ Italy ☐ Japan ☐ Poland ☐ New Zealand ☐ Norway ☐ Western world ☐ Switzerland ☐ Israel ☐ Sweden	☐ UK ☐ China ☐ USA ☐ Spain ☐ Australia ☐ Canada ☐ USA, Canada, UK ☐ Netherlands ☐ Finland ☐ France
Language	☐ English ☐ Chinese ☐ French	☐ German ☐ Italian ☐ other:
Reviewer		
Date		
Exclusion	☐ yes	☐ no
Reason for exclusion		

15

□ Table 15.19 Design, implementation, results, comments

Question	Answer
Objective	☐ health economics ☐ health economics + CAM ☐ usage (reasons, frequency) ☐ safety ☐ exclusion (state reason) free text:...
Participants	☐ physicians ☐ patients (adults, general) ☐ combined (physicians and patients) ☐ population (adults) ☐ patients (adults specific) ☐ patients (children general) ☐ patients (children specific) ☐ patients (adults + children) ☐ population (children)
Study design (category)	☐ literature overview/ meta-analysis ☐ evaluation (quantitative) ☐ cost-effectiveness study ☐ cost-benefit study ☐ cost-of-illness study ☐ cost-minimisation study ☐ evaluation (qualitative)
Design	
Outcomes	
Design (time)	☐ cross-sectional ☐ longitudinal ☐ combined (cross-sectional + longitudinal) ☐ n.a. ☐ not documented
Kind of data	☐ primary data ☐ secondary data ☐ combined (primary + secondary) ☐ n.a. ☐ not documented
Kind of data capture	☐ retrospective ☐ prospective ☐ combined (retrospective + prospective) ☐ n.a. ☐ not documented
Data source (secondary data)	☐ patient records ☐ literature review ☐ n.a. ☐ not documented ☐ other data source

▼

▣ Table 15.19 (continued)

Question	Answer
Questionnaire?	☐ yes ☐ no ☐ n.a. ☐ not documented
Instrument development and validation	
Design of questions	☐ standardized ☐ partly standardized ☐ not standardized ☐ n.a. ☐ not documented ☐ combined (standardized partly and total)
Kind of interview	☐ face to face ☐ telephone interview ☐ paper and pencil ☐ n.a. ☐ not documented
Design, comment and additional information	
Data collection bias	
Indication	
Location/general population	
Sample (description)	
Selection criteria	
Selection bias	
Patient information (diagnosis, age etc.)	
N (number of patients approached)	
Number of patients per group	
Responder (%)	
Non-responder bias	
CAM method (state method investigated)	☐ homeopathy ☐ phytotherapy ☐ TCM ☐ neural therapy ☐ several methods ☐ not documented
Conventional method ▼	if applicable: state method that was investigated or compared

15

◘ Table 15.19 (continued)	
Question	Answer
Results (general)	
CAM: frequency	frequency of usage
CAM: reasons for usage	reasons for usage
CAM: kind of usage	kind of usage
CAM: user profile	CAM user characteristics (as opposed to patients who do not use CAM)
CAM: attitude towards	attitude towards CAM
CAM: effectiveness	perceived effectiveness of CAM
CAM: safety rating	CAM safety rating
CAM: health economic results	
General comments	
n.a.: not applicable	

15.2 Abbreviations

ADHD (=ADHS)	Attention deficit hyperactivity disorder/syndrome
AOK	Allgemeine Ortskrankenkasse (German local insurance provider)
ASA	Acetylsalicylic Acid
AVP	Arzneiverordnung in der Praxis (information brochure published by the Drug Commission of the German Physicians' Association – Arzneimittelkommission der deutschen Ärzteschaft AkdÄ)
BAG	Bundesamt für Gesundheit (Schweiz) – Swiss Federal Office of Health
BGA	Bundesgesundheitsamt (Deutschland) – German Office of Health
BKK	Betriebskrankenkasse (German company sickness insurance fund)
BKK LV NRW	Company sickness insurance fund for the German state of North-Rhine Westphalia
BR	Bundesrat (Swiss Federal Council)
BSE	Bovine spongiform encephalopathy (mad cow disease)
BSV	Bundesamt für Sozialversicherung (Swiss Federal Social Insurance Office FSIO)
CAM	complementary and alternative medicine
CBM	cognition-based medicine
CCT	controlled clinical study
CI	confidence interval (Konfidenzintervall)
CNAMTS	Caisse Nationale d'Assurance Maladie des Travailleurs Salariés
COM	conventional medicine
DAHTA	Deutsche Agentur für Health Technology Assessment (German Agency for Health Technology Assessment)

DIMDI	Deutsches Institut für medizinische Information und Dokumentation (German Institute for medical information and documentation)
DSM IV	Diagnostic and Statistical Manual of Mental Disorders (4th revision)
EBM	Einheitlicher Bewertungsmaßstab Ärzte (German standard fee scale for physicians)
EBM	evidence-based medicine
ECHTA	European Collaboration for Assessment of Health Interventions
EGK	Eidgenössische Gesundheitskasse (Swiss Federal Health Insurance)
ELK	Eidgenössische Kommission für allgemeine Leistungen (Swiss Federal Commission for General Health Insurance)
EMR	Erfahrungsmedizinisches Register (Swiss Register of Empirical Medicine)
EU	European Union
EV	external validity
FEV	forced expiratory volume
FMH	Federatio Medico Helveticorum
FSIO	Swiss Federal Social Insurance Office
GHH	Glasgow Homeopathic Hospital (outcome scale)
GKV	Gesetzliche Krankenversicherung (German Statutory Health Insurance)
GMP	good medical practice
GNP	gross national product
GOÄ/EBM	Gebührenordnung für Ärzte/Einheitlicher Bewertungsmaßstab Ärzte (German medical fee schedule/ standard fee scale physicians)
HAB 2000	Homöopathisches Arzneibuch (German Homeopathic Pharmacopoeia)
HBDT	Human Basophil Degranulation Test
HTA	Health Technology Assessment
IFAEMM	Institut für angewandte Erkenntnistheorie und medizinische Methodologie – Institute for applied epistemology and medical methodology
IIPCOS	International Integrative Primary Care Outcomes Study
IKK	Innungskrankenkasse (German insurance provider)
IKS	Interkantonales Heilmittelinstitut, now: swissmedic (Swiss Agency for Therapeutic Products)
INAHTA	International Network of Agencies for Health Technology Assessment
ISPM	Institut für Sozial- und Präventivmedizin (Institute for social and preventive medicine at Bern University)
ITT	intention to treat (- analysis)
IV	internal validity
KIKOM	Kollegiale Instanz für Komplementärmedizin – Institute for complementary medicine at Bern University
KSK	Konkordat der Schweizerischen Krankenversicherer (now: santésuisse) – Association of Swiss health insurers
KV	Kassenärztliche Vereinigung (German Association of Statutory Health Insurance Physicians)
KVG	Krankenversicherungsgesetz – Swiss Health Insurance Act
LVCF	last value carried forward
MA	meta-analysis
MV	model validity
n.a.	not applicable

NAD	no abnormality detected
n.d. (or nd)	not documented
NFP	Nationales Forschungsprogramm (National Research Programme)
NHS	National Health Service (UK)
NICE	National Institute for Clinical Excellence, UK
NIH	National Institutes of Health (USA)
NRP	National Research Programme
OR	odds ratio
PEK-I	Programm Evaluation Komplementärmedizin, Komponente I (Complementary Medicine Evaluation Programme, component I)
PP	per protocol (- analysis)
RCT	randomized controlled clinical trial
RLHH	Royal London Homeopathic Hospital
SAD	serial agitated dilutions
SAHP	Schweizer Ärztegesellschaft für Homöopathie (Swiss homeopathic physicians' association)
SD	standard deviation
SL	Spezialiäten-Liste (List of specialities)
SPEC	Swiss Patient Care Evaluation Study in Complementary Medicine
SNF	Schweizerischer Nationalfonds (Swiss National Science Foundation)
SNSF	Swiss National Science Foundation
SR	systematic review
SVHA	Schweizerischer Verein Homöopathischer Ärztinnen und Ärzte (Swiss association of homeopathic physicians)
TARMED	tarif médicale
TCM	traditional Chinese medicine
UAE	unexpected adverse event
UK	United Kingdom
UMR/UMK	Unkonventionelle medizinische Richtungen/Unkonventionelle Methoden der Krebsbekämpfung (non-conventional medical approaches, non-conventional cancer therapies)
VAS	visual analogue scale
VSAO	Verband Schweizerischer Assistenz- und Oberärztinnen und -ärzte (Association of Swiss assistant and senior consultants)
WMD	weighted mean difference

15.3   Conflict of interest

Compilation, evaluation and revision of this report were carried out in adherence to the commission documents and the FSIO[1] specification on behalf of the FSIO. Nobody involved in the compilation had any financial or other conflict of interest. Whenever expert advice was sought from a physician who himself uses the method in question, independent experts were also consulted.

15.4   Authors

Klaus von Ammon

Born in Munich in 1955. Human medicine studies in Hamburg, Marburg and Munich 1974–1980; doctorate in 1981. Qualification in neurosurgery in Munich 1981–1988. Consultant and assistant professor at the Department of Neurosurgery, Zurich University Hospital, 1989–1996. Qualification in homeopathy (SVHA/ZAKH, Zurich) from 1997 to 1999. Assistant professor for homeopathy, KIKOM, Bern University since 2000. Medical homeopathic practice near Zurich since 2002. Recognition of homeopathic qualification in 2003.

Address:
Klaus von Ammon, MD
Institute of Complementary Medicine KIKOM, University of Bern
Imhoof-Pavillon, Inselspital, CH-3010 Bern
phone: +41 31 632 97 58
mail: klaus.vonammon@kikom.unibe.ch

Stephan Baumgartner

Born 1965 in Munich. 1984–1990: studies of physics, mathematics and astronomy at Basle University. 1990–1991: research assistant, Section for Mathematics and Astronomy at the Goetheanum in Dornach/Switzerland. 1991–1995: PhD in environmental sciences at the Zurich Institute of Technology (ETH) followed by postdoctoral studies in environmental physics at EAWAG Dübendorf until 1996. Since 1993 Associate at the Department for Fundamental Research, Hiscia Institute, Association for Cancer Research, Arlesheim, and since 1996 also scientific assistant for KIKOM, Bern University.

Address:
Stephan Baumgartner, PhD
Institute of Complementary Medicine KIKOM, University of Bern,
Insel-Spital, Imhoof-Pavillon, CH-3010 Bern
mail: stephan.baumgartner@kikom.unibe.ch

15

---

1   Bundesamt für Sozialversicherung (BSV): Swiss Federal Social Insurance Office

Denise Bloch
Born 1956 in Winterthur/Switzerland. Human medicine studies in Lausanne. Further qualification in general and psychosomatic medicine. Homeopathy training at the Ecole Suisse Romande d'Homéopatie Uniciste in Lausanne, further qualification at the Centre de Santé La Corbière in Estavayer-le-Lac, 1994–1997. Private practice for general and psychosomatic medicine and homeopathy in La Neuveville/CH since 1998.

Address:
Denise Bloch
Chemin du Tirage 21
CH-La Neuveville/BE
phone: +41 32 751 52 67

Gudrun Bornhöft
Born 1959 in Heidelberg. Studies of human medicine in Heidelberg and Kiel 1977–1984. PhD in Kiel 1986. Further specialisation in pathology at the University Hospital Steglitz (now part of the Charité in Berlin) 1985–1993. Lecturer and Director of Studies at Witten/Herdecke University Medical School 1993–1999. Since 2000 assistant professor for Medical Theory and Complementary Medicine.

Address:
Gudrun Bornhöft, MD
Reußstr. 1
D-38640 Goslar
phone: +49 163 62 35 040
mail: gudrun.bornhoeft@online.de

René Gasser
Born 1974 in Naters/Switzerland. Studied sociology at Zurich University 1994–2001. Archivist for SwissRe in Zurich 2001–2002. Worked for WWF (World Wide Fund for Nature) in Schaffhausen/Switzerland 2002–2003. Instructor at the PanMedion Foundation in Zurich 2003–2005.

Peter F. Matthiessen
Born in 1944 in Calw/Wurttemberg, 1964–1971 medical studies at Philipps-University Marburg/Germany and Washington State University St. Louis, 1973 Licensed to practise medicine. 1971–1975 scientific assistant at Marburg University; PhD in 1972. Qualifications in neurology and psychiatry at Herdecke Community Hospital and at the Hospital for Psychiatry Dortmund-Aplerbeck 1975–1980. 1980–1982 Consultant at Marburg University Hospital for Psychiatry; from 1983 Head of Department for Adolescent and Adult Psychiatry at Herdecke Community Hospital. Leading scientist in several research projects, among others: non-conventional medical approaches and non-conventional cancer therapies (UMR/UMK[2]). 1986–1996 directed

---

2   UMR/UMK: Unkonventionelle medizinische Richtungen/ Unkonventionelle Methoden der Krebsbekämpfung (non-conventional medical approaches/ non-conventional cancer therapies)

those two working groups at Witten/Herdecke University under a government mandate to provide an analysis and catalogue of the status of scientific research in CAM; to establish a directed and efficient method of supporting research in CAM; and to coordinate and support various scientific endeavours. 1992 habilitation; from 1997 professorial chair holder for Medical Theory; 2002–2009 professorial holder of the Gerhard-Kienle-Chair for Medical Theory and Complementary Medicine. Since 2009 Head of Department for Plurality of Paradigms in Medicine at Witten/Herdecke University.

Address:
Professor Peter F. Matthiessen, MD, PhD
Zentrum für Integrative Medizin der Universität Witten/Herdecke gGmbH
Gerhard-Kienle-Weg 6
D-58313 Herdecke
phone: +49 2330 62 3890 (secretary: Ulrike Muhr)
fax: +49 2330 62 3358
mail: peter.matthiessen@uni-wh.de

Peter Mattmann
Born 1948, medical studies at Fribourg and Basle. Further qualification in general medicine in Lucerne and various medical practices.
Homeopathy training with Jost Künzli 1985–1988, at August-Weihe-Institut in Detmold and with Alfonso Masi-Elizalde. Lecturer for Oligochrest homeopathy in Switzerland and internationally. PEK-expert homeopathy 2001–2005. Homeopathic private practice in Canton Lucerne since 1977.

Address:
Peter Mattmann-Allamand, MD
Jegerlehnerweg 11
CH-6010 Kriens
phone: +41 41 311 10 15
fax: +41 41 – 311 10 85
mail: mattmann.peter@bluewin.ch

15

Stefanie Maxion-Bergemann
Born 1961 in Esslingen. Studied human medicine in Kiel and Aachen. PhD in Kiel/Germany. Freelance work for medical publishers, since 1988 active in the field of Health Technology Assessment in Germany and Switzerland.

Address:
Stefanie Maxion-Bergemann, MD
Kanderner Str. 39
D-79539 Lörrach
phone: +49 621 910 160
mail: steffi.maxion@gmail.com

Marco Righetti

Born 1953 in Zurich. Medical studies in Zurich 1973–1980, final state examination 1980. Further specialisation in psychiatry-psychotherapy in 1988 and recognition in homeopathy SVHA-FMH. Since 1988 private practice with homeopathic primary care and specialisation in psychiatric-psychosomatic and chronic disease. 1988–2004 president and member of the SVHA training commission. Since 1991 head of SVHA homeopathic training in Zurich. Since 1990 seminars and courses in Germany, Austria and Switzerland. Publications on homeopathy research etc.

Address:
Marco Righetti, MD
Leonhardshalde 2
CH-8001 Zürich
phone +41 44 251 9553

André Thurneysen

Born 1947 in Basle. Medical studies in Zurich, qualification in general medicine FMH and additional qualifications in manual therapy, acupuncture, tropical medicine and classical homeopathy. Since 1980 own practice in Bern/Switzerland, 1995–2008 professorial co-chair holder for classical homeopathy at KIKOM, Bern University. Since 2008 practising in CH-1470 Estavayer-le-Lac.

Address:
André Thurneysen, MD
Centre de Santé La Corbière
CH-1470 Estavayer-le-Lac
phone: +41 26 664 84 20
mail: a.thurneysen@lacorbiere.ch

Christina Vogt-Frank

Born 1961 in Rome. Medical studies in Freiburg and Cologne. Further qualification in general (2001) and psychosomatic medicine (1997). Training in homeopathy from 1991 with recognition of additional title 'homeopathy'. General medical practice since 2003.

Address:
Christina Vogt-Frank
Erlenring 10
D-79540 Stetten Gemeinde Lörrach
phone: +49 7621–49218

Ursula Wolf
Human medicine studies with doctorate and specialist qualification. Biomedical optics research and basic CAM research in USA. Author and co-author for the HTAs of the Swiss PEK programme. Own practice and lecturer and co-director of KIKOM, University of Bern.

Address:
Ursula Wolf, MD
Lecturer, Head of Dept Anthroposophic Medicine
Institute for Complementary Medicine KIKOM
University of Bern
Imhoof-Pavillon, Inselspital
CH-3010 Bern
phone: +41 31 632 97 58
fax: +41 31 632 42 62
mail: ursula.wolf@kikom.unibe.ch

Martin Wolf
Studied electrical engineering at ETH Zurich; doctorate in biomedical technology. Post-doctoral studies at the University of Illinois in Urbana Champaign (physics). At present head of the Biomedical Optics Research Laboratory und lecturer at the University of Zurich.

Address:
Martin Wolf, PhD
Klinik für Neonatologie
Universitätsspital Zürich
Frauenklinikstr. 10
CH-8091 Zürich
phone: +41 44 255 5346
fax:+41 44 – 255 4442
mail: martin.wolf@alumni.ethz.ch

15864927R00136

Printed in Great Britain
by Amazon